ANNUAL REVIEW OF GERONTOLOGY AND GERIATRICS

VOLUME 40, 2020

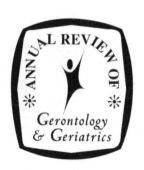

Editors

Series Editor
Roland J. Thorpe, Jr., PhD
Associate Professor
Department of Health, Behavior and Society
Bloomberg School of Public Health
Johns Hopkins University
Baltimore, Maryland

Series Editor and Volume Editor
Jessica A. Kelley, PhD
Professor
Department of Sociology
Case Western Reserve University
Cleveland, Ohio

Annual Review of Gerontology and Geriatrics

Economic Inequality in Later Life

VOLUME 40, 2020

Volume Editor

JESSICA A. KELLEY, PhD

Series Editors

ROLAND J. THORPE, JR., PhD

JESSICA A. KELLEY, PhD

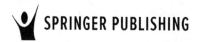

Springer Publishing Company, LLC
11 West 42nd Street,
New York, NY 10036
www.springerpub.com
connect.springerpub.com/

Acquisitions Editor: Adrianne Brigido
Compositor: diacriTech

ISSN: 0198-8794
eISSN: 1944-4036
ISBN: 978-0-8261-4333-4
ebook ISBN: 978-0-8261-4334-1
DOI: 10.1891/9780826143341

20 21 22 / 5 4 3 2 1

The author and the publisher of this Work have made every effort to use sources believed to be reliable to provide information that is accurate and compatible with the standards generally accepted at the time of publication. The author and publisher shall not be liable for any special, consequential, or exemplary damages resulting, in whole or in part, from the readers' use of, or reliance on, the information contained in this book. The publisher has no responsibility for the persistence or accuracy of URLs for external or third-party Internet websites referred to in this publication and does not guarantee that any content on such websites is, or will remain, accurate or appropriate.

Publisher's Note: **New and used products purchased from third-party sellers are not guaranteed for quality, authenticity, or access to any included digital components.**

Contents

About the Volume Editor

Jessica A. Kelley, PhD, is professor and director of the graduate program, Department of Sociology, Case Western Reserve University, Cleveland, Ohio. Dr. Kelley studies the causes and consequences of health disparities over the life course, particularly those related to race, socioeconomic status, and disability. She has expertise in the quantitative analysis of longitudinal and panel data, including latent trajectories and multilevel modeling. Her recent research has focused on life course influences on later-life functional disparities among Black and White adults; how cohort trends and social change affect later-life health profiles; social influences on the experience of disability; neighborhoods and social exclusion of older adults.

Dr. Kelley currently serves as coeditor (with Dr. Roland J. Thorpe, Jr., of Johns Hopkins School of Public Health) of the series *Annual Review of Gerontology and Geriatrics*. She is also Associate Editor of *Journal of Gerontology: Social Sciences* and serves on the Editorial Boards of *Journal of Aging and Health, Research on Aging,* and *Journal of Aging and Social Policy.* Dr. Kelley currently serves on the Advisory Board for the Resource Center for Minority Data at the Interconsortium for Social and Political Research. She also recently completed terms as Chair of the Section on Aging and the Life Course in the American Sociological Association and Member-at-Large for the Behavioral and Social Sciences section of the Gerontological Society of America.

Contributors

Ronald J. Angel, PhD, Professor, Department of Sociology, University of Texas at Austin, Austin, Texas

Deborah Carr, PhD, Professor and Chair, Department of Sociology, Boston University, Boston, Massachusetts

Dale Dannefer, PhD, Selah Chamberlain Professor of Sociology and Chair, Department of Sociology, Case Western Reserve University, Cleveland, Ohio

Marissa Gilbert, MS, Doctoral Student, Department of Sociology, Case Western Reserve University, Cleveland, Ohio

Chengming Han, MS, Doctoral Student, Graduate Research Assistant, Department of Sociology, Case Western Reserve University, Cleveland, Ohio

Katherine Newman, PhD, Interim Chancellor, Office of the Chancellor, Senior Vice President for Academic Affairs, University of Massachusetts Boston, Boston, Massachusetts

Verónica Montes de Oca, PhD, Institute for Social Research of the National Autonomous University of Mexico (UNAM), Senior Researcher, Social Research Institute, Universidad Nacional Autónoma de México, Mexico City, Mexico

Christopher Phillipson, PhD, Manchester Institute for Collaborative Research on Ageing, Professor, Sociology & Social Gerontology, University of Manchester, Manchester, England

Larry Polivka, PhD, Executive Director, Claude Pepper Center on Aging, Florida State University, Tallahassee, Florida

Christian E. Weller, PhD, Professor, Department of Public Policy and Public Affairs, McCormack Graduate School, University of Massachusetts Boston, Boston, Massachusetts

Previous Volumes in the Series

Vol. 29, 2009: Life-Course Perspectives on Late Life Health Inequalities

Editors: Toni C. Antonucci, PhD, and James S. Jackson, PhD

Vol. 28, 2008: Gerontological and Geriatric Education

Editors: Harvey L. Sterns, PhD, and Marie A. Bernard, MD

Vol. 27, 2007: Biopsychosocial Approaches to Longevity

Editors: Leonard W. Poon, PhD, DPhil, and Thomas T. Perls, MD, MPH

Vol. 26, 2006: The Crown of Life Dynamics of the Early Postretirement Period

Editors: Jacquelyn Boone James, PhD, and Paul Wink, PhD

Vol. 25, 2005: Aging Health Care Workforce Issues

Editors: Toni Miles, MD, PhD, and Antonio Furino, PhD, JD

CHAPTER 1

Reconstructing Work and Retirement

Changing Pathways and Inequalities in Later Life

Christopher Phillipson

ABSTRACT

This chapter provides a critical perspective on the reconstruction of work and retirement, as developed through the policy of extending working life. The chapter examines how the idea of extended working lives has been supported by a narrative that disregards concerns about the impact of a "shorter retirement" on groups such as women and blue-collar workers, laying emphasis on older workers as a healthier (and wealthier) group with access to a variety of options for managing the end of working life. The analysis developed suggests that the move to extend working life has run parallel with the emergence of precarious forms of work, with these having major consequences for particular groups such as women and blue-collar workers. The chapter pays particular attention to new forms of insecurity arising from technological changes in the workplace, and the implications of these for supporting longer working lives. The discussion concludes with proposal for reform which could alleviate precarious working translating into precarious forms of retirement. The ideas discussed include: interventions which address inequalities in the workplace; implementing differentiated pathways to retirement; providing enhanced support for women juggling work and care responsibilities; and reassessing the value of the term "older worker."

© 2020 Springer Publishing Company
http://dx.doi.org/10.1891/0198-8794.40.1

INTRODUCTION

The social organization of work and retirement has undergone radical change over the past half century. By the 1960s, retirement had emerged as an established stage in the life course, underpinned in industrial societies by old age insurance and defined benefit pensions (Atchley, 1982). However, the stability of retirement was challenged from the late-1970s onward: initially through the expansion of early retirement or "early exit" (Kohli, Rein, Guillemard, & van Gunsteren, 1991); subsequently, through policies aimed at encouraging longer working lives (Organisation of Economic Cooperation and Development [OECD], 2006; 2019a, 2019b).

Research on work and retirement is now adjusting to an environment influenced by demographic change associated with increased longevity (Gratton & Scott, 2016); technological developments linked with automation in the workplace (Frey, 2019); and economic pressures reflected in job insecurity and underemployment (Blanchflower, 2019). Substantial reviews of work and retirement issues have been produced (e.g., Field, Burke, & Cooper, 2013; Hyde et al., 2018; Wang & Schultz, 2010), supported by analyses of longitudinal data sets from the United States and Europe (e.g., Berkman, Boersch-Supan, & Avendano, 2015; Kendig & Nazroo, 2016; Lain, 2016). Against this, theoretical perspectives in social gerontology have yet to fully engage with social changes, taking place across the majority of industrial countries, driven by rising pension and Social Security ages.

Hasselhorn and Apt (2015, p. 20) refer to the increasing complexity of processes associated with work-ending, in particular the: "[. . .] multilevel and interacting influences of society (macro-level), workplace and organization (meso-level) and the individual (micro-level) on employment participation." A key dimension to the changing relationship between aging and work is the tension between policies to extend working life (EWL)—through the 60s and beyond—and the increasingly fragmented and precarious nature of employment, with the emergence of varied transitions from work to retirement, including: bridge employment, second/third careers, part-time working, "un-retirement," and other variations (see Hasselhorn & Apt, 2015, for definitions of these terms). Such developments indicate both the challenge of conceptualizing new pathways from employment, and—in policy terms—the extent to which these can successfully accommodate longer working lives (James & Pitt-Catsouphes, 2016).

This chapter provides a critical perspective on the reconstruction of work and retirement, as developed through the policy of extending working life. The chapter argues that the idea of longer or extended working lives has been supported by a narrative that disregards concerns about the impact of a "shorter retirement" on groups such as women and blue-collar workers, laying emphasis on older workers as a healthier (and wealthier) group with access to a variety of options for managing the end of working life. To review these issues, the chapter, first, summarizes the various changes affecting the construction of work and retirement; second, outlines a theoretical framework linking precarious work with retirement; third, applies this approach to understanding new inequalities affecting older women and men; and, finally, considers a number of public policy reforms in the area of extending working life.

Changing Pathways From Work to Retirement

Understanding those factors that determine whether older workers remain in their current employment, take partial retirement, return to work, or retire completely, has developed as an important topic of study within social gerontology (Kojola & Moen, 2016). Research in this area suggests an interplay between the state, organizations, and individuals influencing transitions from work to retirement (Laczko & Phillipson, 1991; Macnicol, 2015; Vickerstaff, 2006), with three main periods identified in the research literature: first, the emergence of retirement in the 1950s and 1960s; second, the expansion of early retirement in the 1970s and 1980s; third, the "individualization" of retirement, along with pressures to extend working life, from the late-1990s and continuing. The first phase occurred in the two decades following the ending of the Second World War, notably with the development (in Europe) of the welfare state together with the application (across most industrial countries) of mandatory retirement (Atchley, 1982; Graebner, 1980). Both were instrumental in shaping the discourse around which old age was constructed over the course of the 1950s and 1960s (Phillipson, 2019).

The idea of "retirement" was a central part of the narrative driving the reconstruction of aging, with Vickerstaff (2015, p. 298) highlighting its role in creating a "predictable, age-patterned end to working life." However, the institution of retirement was itself destabilized by rising levels of unemployment and redundancies, beginning in the 1960s but accelerating through the 1970s and 1980s (Kohli et al., 1991). To take one example, in 1971, 83% of men 60 to 64 in the United Kingdom were in employment, compared with 19% of those 65 plus; by 1981 the figures had declined to 69% and 10%; and by 1991 to 54% and 10% (Phillipson, 2013).

The trends identified established a new phase in the relationship between work and retirement, with researchers drawing a distinction between "retirement" on the one side and "early exit" on the other: the former referring to entry into a publicly-provided old-age pension scheme; the latter, early withdrawal from paid employment supported through unemployment, disability, or associated benefits. Guillemard and van Gunsteren (1991, p. 383) argued that the consequence of these changes was a life course that was ". . . becoming variable, imprecise, and contingent, since chronological milestones [were] being torn up." The decades of the 1970s and 1980s brought significant changes in attitudes toward work and retirement. The image of retirement was transformed, with a shift toward "viewing it as an eagerly anticipated escape from the routine of work to the discretion of leisure" (Hardy, 2011, p. 215). Arguments emerged suggesting that an extended period of retirement could lead to more expansive lifestyles, these reflected in the activities of the baby boom generation now entering their fifties and sixties (Gilleard & Higgs, 2005). Hyde et al. (2018, p. 13) argue that during the 1980s retirement went from being seen as a "bleak, depressing stage of life to being seen as a time for enjoyment, adventure, personal growth and fulfilment after a lifetime of work. [Such] ideas coincided with falling rates of labor market participation in later life as many people took advantage of opportunities for early retirement."

Policies toward work and retirement changed once again during the 1990s and into the 2000s, with concerns raised about the potential economic and social costs of population aging (OECD, 2006). On the one side came pressure on individuals to remain in some form of work for as long as possible; on the other side a decline in the institutional supports associated with the welfare state. These developments were underpinned by, first, increases in pension ages in many OECD countries; second, a reduction in options to retire "early" on grounds of ill health; third, reductions in disability benefits. These factors increased the reliance of individuals on the market (and employment), with emphasis placed on the responsibility of individuals to manage their own retirement and preferably to delay leaving work for as long as possible (Hofäcker, Hess, & König, 2016; König, Hess, & Hofäcker, 2016; Lain, 2016; Macnicol, 2015; Nì Léime & Loretto, 2017).

Social Institutions and Work-Ending
The periods identified produced variations in the balance of social institutions influencing work-ending. In the first—from the 1950s through to the end of the 1960s—the state was dominant, reflecting the role of mandatory retirement and welfare provision regulating the passage from paid employment through to retirement (Kohli et al., 1991). Employers played an important, albeit secondary, role, illustrated by the growth (mostly for men) of defined benefit pension schemes (Hannah, 1986), in enabling continued employment (largely for men in their sixties), and in the development of preretirement education—an area of interest in the United Kingdom and United States in the 1950s and 1960s (Glamser, 1981; Phillipson, 1981). During the 1970s and 1980s the state and employers played

a more equal role shaping transitions from work to retirement. The state exercised influence in setting out the terms of the response to the challenge of finding employment for a large cohort of younger workers. Early retirement came to be viewed as a "bloodless" (Kohli et al., 1991, p. 11) way of coping with structural unemployment in industries such as mining and steel. But employers were crucial in the development of measures to facilitate early retirement and other pathways from employment. As a result, much of the decision-making power in the 1980s about retirement rested neither with the state nor with individuals but shifted to the discretion of employers (Guillemard & van Gunsteren, 1991). Individuals (mainly men in white-collar occupations) had some control over whether to stay at work or leave employment, especially if supported by an occupational pension. But the decline in employment in many industrial countries suggests pressure to leave work, even if for some early retirement was an attractive prospect given the burden associated with many forms of employment (Sennett & Cobb, 1977).

From the 1990s onward, all three actors—the state, employers, and individuals—became involved in shaping work–retirement transitions. The general context was one of governments encouraging people to work longer while shifting the burden of paying for a longer life onto the shoulders of individuals (Macnicol, 2015; Weller, 2016). At the same time, moves to extend working life increased the influence of employers, for example in determining (late) career options; supporting flexible/partial retirement; and facilitating job redesign. For older workers, entering what Vickerstaff (2006, p. 509) defined as the "retirement zone," the ability to control "work-ending" was subject to variation according to class, gender, health, occupation, and related factors. Wang, Olson, and Schultz (2013, p. 7) suggest that some late career workers at least have ". . . increased freedom and choice and also have the resources to make personal choices and search for self-fulfilment." However, organizational pressures associated with downsizing and technological change limited career options for many, increasing the importance of supporting employees entering their fifties and sixties (Wang et al., 2013).

The present context facing older workers has a number of unique features: governments appear set on policies to extend working lives; employers are at early stage of adjusting to a relatively new demographic and labor market context; and older workers themselves are facing an "uncertain future" in reconciling pressures associated with longer working, combined with job and pension insecurity (Wainwright et al., 2019). Henkens et al. (2018, p. 806) conclude that: "The social and economic transformations surrounding retirement are generally expected to be characterized by longer lives, greater uncertainty and inequality surrounding public pension rights and levels, and the need to assume greater labour market and savings risks over the [life course]." Such changes led McDonald and Donahue (2011, p. 414) to conclude that retirement as a social institution had been abandoned in the race to raise pension and Social Security ages.

The developments identified suggest the potential "break-up" or "fragmentation" of two major social institutions: employment on the one side; retirement on the other. In the former case, this has been driven by major changes in the workplace leading to increasingly precarious forms of working (see the following), along with the move to extend working life. But this has also translated into a more "fragmented" form of retirement, with contrasting opportunities according to gender, class, and minority group status. The next section of this chapter reviews the theoretical context for this development, drawing on theories which have identified the emergence of greater insecurity and "precariousness" within the labor markets of Western economies.

Precarious Work and Retirement

A central argument of this chapter is that the development of policies to lengthen working lives—facilitated by changes to occupational and state pension systems—coincided with the onset of "precarious" forms of employment affecting labor markets in industrial economies. Kalleberg (2018, p. 201) suggests that:

> The idea of precarious work has gained wide currency among social theorists as a way of describing the condition of growing insecurity and uncertainty in contemporary capitalism that results from processes of globalization, technological change, the weakening of workers' power, and the political and cultural dynamics associated with neoliberalism . . . This growth of precarious work represents a partial return to the market-mediated employment systems and relative lack of social protections that preceded the development of the Keynesian welfare state, and has created considerable uncertainty and insecurity about the future of jobs and careers . . . .

Standing (2011) links the growth of precarious forms of work to the impact of globalization and the fragmentation of traditional class identities (see, further, Savage, 2015). This he views as producing a distinctive social group —the "precariat"—one which lacks various forms of labor-related security, including: labor market security, for example, adequate income-earning opportunities; employment security, for example, protection against arbitrary dismissal; and income security, for example, assurance of an adequate stable income. Standing (2011) argues that a range of groups have joined the precariat, including women, ethnic minorities, and older people, with the last of these taking low-level jobs in later life, largely to supplement inadequate pensions and/or health insurance. Accordingly, certain groups of older people can find themselves in a "precarity trap," forced to remain or reenter the workforce in flexible and lower-income status positions. Older people with limited financial resources may themselves rely upon precarious workers as carers, and family networks may be reduced or drained by means of their own precarity (see, further, Lain, Airey, Loretto, & Vickerstaff, 2019)

The growth of precarious working might be further viewed as a consequence of the type of work–retirement transitions which developed from the 1990s. These entailed a loosening of retirement (and associated rites of passage) on the one side; and a weakening of supports provided through the welfare state on the other side. The assumption was that workers were entering a new period of choice and control, "reinventing retirement" as a time where different combinations of work and leisure-orientated activities could be developed (Altmann, 2015). This was itself seen as fueled by the rise of the baby-boom cohort, a group viewed as wanting a greater range of employment-related options in comparison with earlier cohorts (Lain et al., 2019).

But the development of precarious employment complicates the idea of later-life working constructed around a great degree of choice, underpinned by different forms of flexible employment. An alternative view would see this environment as an extension of Beck's (1992) "risk society," with retirement reverting to a "social risk" rather than a "social right," but with the idea that encouraging longer working lives—through raising pension ages—can provide a secure bridge into older age. But the extent to which work is becoming *more* rather than *less* secure, raises problems for this approach. Taylor (2019) makes the point that the terms of an individual's labor market engagement is of critical importance. Yet, as he notes: "Many older people move into bridge forms of employment in contingent, non-core areas of the labor market with the attendant risks of poor health and injury associated with poor work organization, and a lack of adequate training" (Taylor, 2019, p. 101). Moreover, "rather than acknowledge the potential health and other risks associated with poor-quality, precarious or unwanted work, emerging narratives of working longer from a healthy aging perspective have generally ignored such issues" (Taylor, 2019, p. 101).

Precarious Working and Technological Change

A further issue affecting the reconstruction of work and retirement, concerns the impact of technological development and the influence of automation in the workplace. Caution is needed in respect of judgments about the type and rate of change. However, it is clear that at least in respect of the immediate future facing workers (especially those unskilled and semiskilled), industrial change is likely to be both intensive and extensive—not least in those areas which have borne the brunt of deindustrialization (Frey, 2019). The development of EWL has in fact come at a time when "good quality" employment appears to be contracting through a range of processes affecting the workplace (Avent, 2016; Frey, 2019; Srnicek & Williams, 2015). This may be less an issue for the *existing* cohort of employed older workers, notably those in long-term employment. However, EWL is being implemented when opportunities for full-time employment in later life are *contracting*—illustrated by the decline in labor force participation among prime age workers, the sharp decline in the share of workers employed in manufacturing, and the impact of "underemployment" (Benanav, 2019; Blanchflower, 2019; Dvorkin & Shell, 2015). Instead, there is the growth of employment with limited security in respect of pensions, health insurance, and guaranteed hours (Srnicek & Williams, 2015; Weller, 2016): employment which may be increasingly targeted at older workers displaced from their main careers (Lain et al., 2019; Standing, 2011).

In the United Kingdom, much of the job growth among older workers has consisted of self-employment (accounting for nearly one in two workers aged 65-plus), but with this typically producing low levels of income for those entering or remaining in this type of work. In the United States, a survey by Koenig, Trawinski, and Rix (2015) found that those aged 45 to 70 who had been unemployed in the past 5 years and who were reemployed were twice as likely to be working part-time as the total workforce in this age group: 34% compared with 16%. Equally significant was the finding that 48% of those who had found new jobs said that they were now earning less when compared with the job they had before becoming unemployed.

To what extent will changes to employment increase or decrease the demand for older workers? One neglected area in EWL policy is the degree to which technological change is likely to change the terms of the debate about the extent to which later life employment can be achieved. Frey and Osborne (2013) predict in the case of the United States that 47% of jobs are at "high risk" of being automated in the next decade, with similar estimates being made for Europe (Frey & Osborne 2015). These authors make the point that while new technology can both generate as well as destroy jobs, the former tend to be rather fewer than the latter, noting that: "In 2010 only about 0.5 percent of the U.S. workforce was employed in new industries that did not exist a decade earlier" (Frey & Osborne, 2015, p. 63). Importantly, most of these jobs were at the high skill/high education/high wage end, suggesting limited job growth in areas which might fit an increased supply of older workers. Frey (2019, p. 350) further suggests that while "unskilled work is not coming to an end . . . low skilled jobs [are likely to be] more exposed to future automation."

Overall, it may well be the case that jobs will continue to be produced to sustain longer working lives; but the nature of these remains uncertain, with evidence for a rise in job insecurity and fear of unemployment affecting particular countries and groups of workers (Blanchflower, 2019). The OECD (2019a) calculate that only a minority of jobs (14%) are at *high risk* of automation. But automation is unlikely to affect people and places in equal ways. The United Kingdom Office for National Statistics (2019b) examined changes over the period 2011 to 2017 in the risk of automation, finding a slight *decline* over the period in people employed in jobs at high risk of automation (7.4% in 2017; against 8.1% in 2011). Importantly, though, when looking at those in jobs classed as "high risk," women accounted for 70.2% of employees (reflecting changes in retail and administrative jobs); compared with women accounting for 42.6% of employees at low risk of automation. Also of note was the finding that the risk of automation increased with the age group 40 to 44 years and upwards (see, also, Rutledge, Wettstein, & King, 2019).

Inequality and Precarious Work-Endings

The trends discussed in the previous section are of considerable importance given the move to raise pension and Social Security ages as a means of extending working life (or discouraging retirement). Over the course of the 1990s and into the opening decades of the 2000s, a majority of OECD countries implemented a range of pension reforms, key to which were raising the age at which pensions could be drawn—typically from 65 to 67 but with later ages also planned (Axelrad & Mahoney, 2017). This was also linked with the abolition of mandatory retirement in a number of countries, giving people the theoretical right to continue working into their sixties, seventies, and beyond. At the same time, as Loretto and Vickerstaff (2015, p. 176) observe: "Very little [was] typically said about the differential capacity of people to work or the . . . neglected question of whether there [was] sufficient labour market demand to absorb extended working lives." Indeed, an emerging issue is precisely the extent to which a new "zone of insecurity" has developed for people in their fifties and sixties, with increasing numbers stranded without access to suitable employment but deemed too young to draw a pension.

The OECD (2019b) report that in 26 (out of 36) member countries, one-quarter of men still retired below the age of 60 in 2018, with the corresponding age often substantially lower in the case of women. While average effective retirement age (ERA) has risen in a majority of OECD countries since the late-1990s, it is still below the level in 1980 in most (see, further, OECD, 2017). This suggests that delaying the point at which pensions can be drawn until people are in their late sixties (or seventy before full Social Security benefits are available in the case of the United States) is likely to cause considerable hardship for many groups struggling to retain a hold in the labor market. This is especially true in the case of women (see the following) where the average gender gap in OECD countries stood at 18% for 55 to 64 years olds in 2018, down by only 3% points from 2008 (OECD, 2019a, 2019b).

The experience of the United Kingdom is illustrative of the pressures affecting people faced with working longer in the context of precarious labor markets. Lain et al. (2019, p. 2225) argues that the United Kingdom is moving toward what they term "a 'self-reliance' model where most individuals now have the theoretical right to continue working past 65, but [with] rapid State Pension age increases [offering] little realistic alternative to employment." State pension ages for both sexes will increase to 66 by 2020 and 67 in 2028, with regular reviews thereafter. But despite much being made of progress in achieving longer work lives (Department for Work and Pension [DWP], 2017), a different picture emerges from examining trends in the average age of exit from the labor market (i.e., the age at which people over 50 are most likely to leave the labor force). In the case of men, a high point was reached soon after the Second World War, with an average age of exit in 1950 of 67.2 years. The trend thereafter was downward to a low of 63.0 (in 1996), with increases thereafter but with virtually no movement since 2016 (65.2); 65.3 years in 2019. The figures for women have been influenced by the equalization of pension ages, with the average age of exit in 2019 64.3 years, compared with a previous high in 1950 of 63.9 years (DWP, 2019). Men's average age of exit increased by just 12 months in the 11 years from 2008 to 2019. Leaving aside the exceptional years of full employment in a postwar economy, the average age of exit for men has fluctuated between 63 and 65 (for women 62 and 64) over a period of 60 years, but in a period characterized by a decline in the type of employment (i.e., manufacturing) which sustained blue-collar employment and the entry of women into different forms of (largely) part-time work.

The figures presented suggest that, at least taking the example of the United Kingdom, extending working life into the late sixties and early seventies will produce new inequalities at the end of working life, in particular for groups such as women, workers from minority groups, and those in poor health. The extent of inequality arising from EWL, and the rapid reversal from early retirement, has been documented in a series of studies, notably in Germany, but also other European countries, for example, those by Rinklake and Buchholz (2011), Buchholz, Rinklake, and Blossfield (2013), Hofäcker and Naumann (2015), and Hofäcker, Hess, and Naumann (2015). Hofäcker and Naumann (2015) make the point that early exit pathways, as developed in the 1970s and 1980s, were an important route for workers with low or limited skills, reducing the financial penalty associated with the loss of work. Closure of these pathways, however, has forced many to continue working longer—but mainly driven by financial need rather than any active choice to remain in the labor market. Hofäcker et al. (2015, p. 223) conclude from their survey of the labor market situation of older workers in 30 countries (drawing on data from the European Social Survey), that

> [. . .] recent policy developments create new risks such as old age poverty that mainly threaten low-skilled workers [. . .] As a result of anticipated benefit cuts for early pension entrance, these workers have to continue working although their chances of finding an adequate job is comparably low—either because of their individual health or because of their critical labour market situation.

Lain (2016, pp. 138–140) makes the point that financial, rather than intrinsic or social reasons for working are *higher* among the poorest segments of the workforce than the richest, and highest among those with poor levels of health and/education. Analysis of workers aged 65 to 67 in the 2008 U.S. Health and Retirement Survey found that 84.2% of those in the poorest wealth quartile said they would like to stop working but needed the money, with similar proportions saying the same thing among with those below high school qualifications and those in poor/fair health. Lain and Phillipson (2019) argue, on the basis of this and other research, that it is reasonable to conclude that many individuals continue working even though they view it as being detrimental to their health and well-being.

GENDER, PRECARITY, AND LATER LIFE WORKING

The emphasis on lengthening working lives has raised particular concerns for groups such as older women, given continuing gender inequalities both at work and at home (Lewis, 2006). Street (2017, p. 22) makes the point that women earn less for equivalent jobs, are more likely to take a career break to care for children, and to care for a disabled adult child and older family members. Such factors underline the dangers of raising pension ages in the absence of a broader set of policies designed to support women (and men) at different phases of the life course. Implementation of EWL, however, would suggest that public concerns have been viewed as secondary to the broader issue of responding to pressures arising from population aging (Nì Léime & Ogg, 2019). Nì Léime and Loretto (2017, p. 58) highlight the extent to which women are presented as an "untapped labor reserve," able to fill the job vacancies arising from population aging. But the research literature, as summarized in the following, highlights a number of difficulties with this argument, raising concerns about the extent to which women will be able to keep working through their sixties and beyond.

First, there is the tension between normative assumptions about women as primary carers and the move to extend working lives (Della Guista & Jewell, 2015). The OECD (e.g., 2017), in their regular series of reports on pension trends, highlight contrasting reasons for exit from the labor market reported by women and men: the former most likely ceasing paid work to care for other family members; the latter via retirement or through unemployment or disability. In the United Kingdom, almost one in four (24%) of female workers have caring responsibilities, as compared with one in eight (13%) of male workers (Office for National Statistics [ONS], 2019a). Loretto and Vickerstaff (2015) argue that this aspect of women's work (often centered around caring for parents and grandchildren) has gone unrecognized in debates around extending working life, amplifying inequalities within the domestic sphere. Harrington Meyer's (2014) study of working grandmothers explored the extent to which intensive caregiving followed women into the fifties, sixties, and seventies. Notwithstanding the rewards associated with grandparenting, Harrington Meyer pointed to some of the challenges facing grandmothers juggling work and care, including financial constraints of intensive grandmothering; the difficulties women experience in setting limits on their caregiving; and the lack of understanding from male partners and co-workers. Such pressures are likely to be reinforced through the crisis in social care, with cut-backs in home and day-care services (Kröger & Bagnato, 2018), and the emergence of what (Estes, Swan, & Associates, 1993) termed "no care zones."

Second, there is evidence to suggest that raising pension ages, in the context of managing care responsibilities with longer than expected periods of employment, may have damaging effects on the mental and physical health of some groups of women. Various research studies have suggested that increasing pension ages results in negative physical and mental health outcomes for women (De Grip, Lindeboom, & Montizaan, 2012; Zhu & He, 2015; see, further, Bebbington, 2019). Research in the United Kingdom by Carrino, Glaser, and Avendano (2018) examined the health consequences for women of the raising of state pension age. State pensions contribute to around 45% of the incomes of older people in the United Kingdom, hence any delay in receiving a pension, without alternative sources of support, may have a damaging impact on economic and social well-being. The researchers analyzed a sample of 3,452 women aged 60 to 64 interviewed between 2009 and 2015 as part of Understanding Society, a nationally representative survey with extensive health measures. Carrino et al. (2018, p. 4) report: "strong evidence that an increase in [pension ages] leads to a significant worsening of mental health: UK women no longer eligible to collect their pension at age 60 to 62 as a result of [pension reforms have] worse mental health and higher depression scores than women able to collect their pensions at the same age." The evidence from the research also suggested greater impacts on health for women from routine/manual occupations as opposed to those from the professional sector (see, also, Lain et al., 2019).

Third, findings on the negative health consequences of raising pension ages are especially serious given continuing discrimination in the design of occupational and state pension systems. Nì Léme and Loretto (2017, p. 53) make the point that: "Most pension systems were designed for a male breadwinner model of family life and, as such, did not acknowledge the unpaid caring work usually done by women, which reduced their ability to qualify for or contribute to pensions." Moreover, pension reforms which increase the amount of contributions and switch to lifetime earnings also disadvantage women, who will invariably have had shorter careers and lower earning levels in comparison with men (Arcanjo, 2019).

CONCLUSION

This chapter has argued that the move to extend working life has run parallel with the emergence of precarious forms of work, with these having major consequences for particular groups such as women and unskilled and semiskilled workers. The challenge therefore is how to prevent precarious working lives resulting in precarious retirements (Wall & Abiom, 2016). In general, this is not an issue addressed in mainstream public policy. Pension ages have been moved upwards on the basis of (a) what is seen as an urgent need to control costs; and (b) because lengthy retirements are viewed as a means of promoting "active" and "successful" aging (Street & Tompkins, 2018). But delaying access to pensions and benefits raises serious issues for groups without alternative means of support. In the future, many older workers will remain stranded in a "zone of insecurity" in their fifties to seventies, faced with declining incomes on the one side, and limited job opportunities on the other.

What are the options for public policy, given the tensions identified between a precarious work environment and longer working lives? First, interventions which address insecurities within the workplace will be essential if the policy of EWL is to be maintained. Evidence for the deteriorating quality of the workplace environment—driven by globalization and technological change—is now substantial (see, for example, Smeaton & White, 2016, for United Kingdom evidence on this issue). And the question of whether sufficient jobs will be available in the future is a critical issue to examine when considering the implications of raising pension ages. Based on evidence cited in this chapter, advancing retirement ages in the absence of secure forms of employment is likely to result in an extension of inequalities from the middle to later phases of the life course.

One response may be to recognize that EWL will almost certainly contribute to the *expansion* of "precarious" forms of working but to match this with corresponding *employment rights* (e.g., for those in sectors affected by technological change, for workers experiencing changing conditions of employment), through, for example, ensuring access to trade unions, minimum wages, guaranteed hours, and access to regular training (see Standing, 2014, for a development of this theme).

Second, and following the preceding argument, greater attention needs to be given to the way in which the raising of pension ages is generating inequalities linked to contrasting experiences in terms of health, finances, and social relationships. Many groups of workers are unlikely to benefit from a lengthy period of retirement (dying prematurely) or will have insufficient income to be able to leave what may be "precarious work" in their sixties/early seventies. Others may choose to leave early or have a minimal EWL (because they have substantial pensions and savings) and will experience an active retirement supported by many years of "healthy life expectancy." This indicates new inequalities arising from longer working lives, with a redistribution of resources from the poor to the wealthy. The argument here is for a work and retirement policy which recognizes processes of cumulative advantage and disadvantage operating over the life course (Dannefer, 2003; Kendig & Nazroo, 2016). This point has been made by Berkman et al. (2015, pp. 44–45) where they argue that given divisions between groups (especially in terms of health):

> . . . it is critical to create differentiated paths to retirement and labor-force exits depending upon health (which in turn depends on economic and social experiences earlier in life) . . . This may mean the implementation of both a general retirement age that is indexed in some way to life expectancy and an early-retirement option based on the ability to work. For older workers in poor health, it is obviously better for their health and well-being not to have to work. This may mean that certain groups within the population—such as the less educated and those with very physically demanding jobs—may need the option to take an early path to retirement.

This is an important argument which if adopted could do much to resolve many of the problems associated with the EWL approach. The available evidence, however, suggests that the reverse is happening in many countries, with those in poor health often forced to remain in work to secure health insurance or retirement benefits (Benjamin, Pransky, & Savageau, 2008); or those with a lifetime of low incomes needing to work later in contrast to those with the benefit of secure occupational pensions and/or access to income from property who are able to take early retirement.

Third, as already argued in this chapter, there is a particular tension developing between EWL policies, and pressures on women undertaking care responsibilities in later life. Nì Léme and Loretto (2017, pp. 58–59) suggest that the "individualised adult worker model has meant more work for women, who have tended to add paid work to existing care responsibilities, while men in many Western countries have decreased their amount of paid work, but only slightly increased care." This situation needs an urgent response in terms of action from employers and from public policy more generally. Relevant policies that will need to be implemented across all OECD countries pursuing EWL include: carer's benefits to give paid leave and pension/Social Security credits for time spent caring for older people; public provision for child care and elder care; and policies encouraging men to take a more equitable share in the unpaid work of caring (see, further, Vickerstaff et al., 2017).

Fourth, if retirement is now viewed as a 20th century institution, the same might be said of the term "older workers." Women, men, different ethnic groups, those in growing/declining cities/industries, may have the category fifty plus in common, but very little else which carries sociological meaning. As suggested earlier in this chapter, the "fragmentation" of the label "older worker" can be viewed as the reverse side of the fragmentation of retirement. For some groups, EWL will be a positive addition to an "active aging"; for the "losers from globalization" (Buchholz et al., 2009; men with limited skills, some minority ethnic groups, those living in postindustrial cities), EWL has limited salience as a way of managing "work-ending." In addition, it is possible the term "older worker" itself compounds the problems facing people struggling to remain in work, with research indicating that the moment someone becomes categorized as an "older worker" they are potential targets for prejudice and discrimination (Desmette & Gaillard, 2008).

Finally, whether viewed as a "fuller" or an "extended" working life, it is clear that considerable opportunities exist for rethinking theories concerning the transition from work to retirement. In particular, the evolving landscape raises a challenge to the popularity of rational choice theories which emphasize the power of individuals to choose among different options about their future (e.g., Hofäcker et al., 2016). Vickerstaff and Cox (2005, p. 92) view this as part of the "individualization of retirement," the result of which has been "less to increase the majority of people's range of alternatives and choices over when and how to retire and more to enlarge the range of risks they [have] to cope with." Similarly, Wang and Schultz (2010, p. 186) emphasize the extent to which: ". . . retirement decisions are often made in the face of incomplete and imperfect information, which renders a sense of uncertainty in the decision-making process." They further note that: "So far, no theoretical framework has incorporated this notion of uncertainty, which could have important theoretical implications for understanding the psychological aspect of the retirement decision." However, as the trends surveyed in this chapter suggest, "uncertainty" and "risk" are now a key feature of transitions from mid-life onward (Vickerstaff, 2006, p. 2015). The changes associated with this development reinforce the need for theories and policies alert to the unstable foundations on which the institutions of work and retirement now rest.

REFERENCES

Altmann, R. (2015). *A new vision for older workers: Retain, retrain, recruit*. London, England: Department for Work and Pensions.

Arcanjo, M. (2019). Retirement pension reforms in six European social insurance schemes between 2000 and 2017: More financial sustainability and more gender inequality. *Social Policy & Society*, 18(4), 501–515. https://doi.org/10.1017/S1474746418000398

Atchley, R. (1982). Retirement as a social institution. *Annual Review of Sociology*, 8, 263–287. https://doi.org/10.1146/annurev.so.08.080182.001403

Avent, R. (2016). *The wealth of humans: Work and its absence in the twenty-first century*. London, England: Allen Lane.

Axelrad, H., & Mahoney, K. (2017). Increasing the pensionable age: What changes are OECD countries making? What considerations are driving policy? *Open Journal of Social Sciences*, 5, 56–70. https://doi.org/10.4236/jss.2017.57005

Bebbington, D. (2019). You know something is wrong when your grandmother starts protesting: The impact of the rise in State Pension age on women in UK. *Women's Studies International Forum*, 75, Article 102235. https://doi.org/10.1016/j.wsif.2019.05.004

Beck, U. (1992). *Risk society: Towards a new modernity*. London, England: Sage.

Benanav, A. (2019). Automation and the future of work -1. *New Left Review*, 119, 5–38.

Benjamin, K., Pransky, G., & Savageau, J. A. (2008). Factors associated with retirement-related job lock in older workers with recent occupational injury. *Disability Rehabilitation*, 30, 1976–1983. https://doi.org/10.1080/09638280701772963

Berkman, L., Boersch-Supan, A., & Avendano, M. (2015). Labor force participation, policies and practices in an aging America: Adaptation essential for a healthy & resilient population.d.aedalus. *Journal of the American Academy of Arts & Sciences*, 144, 41–54. doi:10.1162/DAED_a_00329

Blanchflower, D. (2019). *Not working: Where have all the good jobs gone?* Princeton, NJ: Princeton University Press.

Buchholz, S., Hofäcker, D., Mills, M., Blossfeld, H.-F., Kurz, K., & Hofmeister, H. (2009). Life courses in the globalization process: The development of social inequalities in modern societies. *European Sociological Review*, 25, 53–71. https://doi.org/10.1093/esr/jcn033

Buchholz, S., Rinklake, A., & Blossfeld, H.-P. (2013). Reversing early retirement in Germany: A longitudinal analysis of the effects of recent pension reforms on the timing of the transition to retirement and on pension incomes. *Comparative Population Studies, 38*, 881–906.

Carrino, L., Glaser, K., & Avendano, M. (2018). *Later pension, poorer health? Evidence from the new state pension age in the UK* (Working paper series). Cambridge, MA: Harvard University, Harvard Centre for Population and Development.

Dannefer, D. (2003). Cumulative advantage/disadvantage and the life course: Cross fertilizing age and social science theory. *Journal of Gerontology: Social Sciences, 58*(6), S327–S337. https://doi.org/10.1093/geronb/58.6.S327

De Grip, A., Lindeboom, M., & Montizaan, R. (2012). Shattered dreams: The effects of changing the pension system late in the game. *The Economic Journal, 122*(559), 1–25. https://doi.org/10.1111/j.1468-0297.2011.02486.x

Della Guista, M., & Jewell, S. (2015). Unpaid work and conformity: Why care? *Cambridge Journal of Economics, 39*(3), 689–710. https://doi.org/10.1093/cje/beu061

Department for Work and Pensions. (2017). *Fuller working lives: A partnership approach.* London, England: Author.

Department for Work and Pensions. (2019). *Economic labour market status of individuals aged 50 and over, trends over time: September 2019.* London, England: Author.

Desmette, D., & Gaillard, M. (2008). When a 'worker' becomes an 'older worker': The effects of age-related social identity on attitudes towards work and retirement. *Career Development International, 13*(2), 168–195. https://doi.org/10.1108/13620430810860567

Dvorkin, M., & Shell, M. (2015). *Labor force participation: The U.S. and its peers. Federal Bank of St. Louis.* Retrieved from https://www.stlouisfed.org/on-the-economy/2015/june/labor-forceparticipation-the-us-and-its-peers

Estes, C. L., Swan, J. H., and Associates. (1993). *The long-term care crisis: Elders trapped in the no-care zone.* Newbury Park, CA: Sage.

Field, J., Burke, R. J., & Cooper, C. L. (Eds.). (2013). *The Sage handbook of aging work and society.* London, England: Sage.

Frey, C. B. (2019). *The technology trap: Capital, labor, and power in the age of automation.* Princeton, NJ: Princeton University Press.

Frey, C. B., & Osborne, M. (2013). *The future of employment.* Oxford, UK: Oxford Martin School, University of Oxford.

Frey, C. B., & Osborne, M. (2015). *Technology at work: The future of innovation and employment.* Oxford, UK: Oxford Martin School, University of Oxford.

Gilleard, C., & Higgs, P. (2005). *Contexts of ageing: Class, cohort and community.* Cambridge, UK: Polity Press.

Glamser, F. (1981). The impact of the pre-retirement programs on the retirement experience. *Journal of Gerontology, 36*(2), 244–250. https://doi.org/10.1093/geronj/36.2.244

Graebner, W. (1980). *A history of retirement: The meaning and function of an American institution, 1885-1978.* New Haven, CT: Yale University Press.

Gratton, L., & Scott, L. (2016). *The 100 year life: Living and working in an age of longevity*. London, England: Bloomsbury.

Guillemard, A-M., & van Gunsteren, H. (1991) Pathways and their prospects: A comparative interpretation of the meaning of early exit. In M. Kohli, M. Rein, A-M. Guillemard, & H. van Gunsteren (Eds), *Time for retirement: Comparative studies of early exit from the labor force* (pp. 362–388). Cambridge, UK: Cambridge University Press.

Hannah, L. (1986). *Inventing retirement*. Cambridge, UK: Cambridge University Press.

Hardy, M. (2011). Rethinking retirement. In R. Settersten & J. Angel (Eds.), *Handbook of sociology of aging* (pp. 213–228). New York, NY: Springer Publishing.

Harrington Meyer, M. (2014). *Grandmothers at work: Juggling families and jobs*. New York, NY: New York University Press.

Hasselhorn, H. M., & Apt, W. (Eds.). (2015). *Understanding employment: Creating a knowledge base for future labour market challenges*. Berlin, Germany: Federal Ministry of Labour and Social Affairs.

Henkens, K., Dalen van, H., Ekerdt, D., Hershey, D., Hyde, M., Radl, J., & . . . Zacher, H. (2018). What we need to know about retirement: Pressing issues for the coming decade. *Gerontologist, 58*(5), 805–812. https://doi.org/10.1093/geront/gnx095

Hofäcker, D., Hess, M., & König, S. (Eds.). (2016). *Delaying retirement: Progress and challenges of active ageing in Europe, the United States and Europe*. London, England: Palgrave Macmillan.

Hofäcker, D., Hess, M., & Naumann, E. (2015). Changing retirement transitions in times of paradigmatic political change: Towards growing inequalities. In C. Torp (Ed.), *Challenges of ageing* (pp. pp. 205–226). London, England: Palgrave Macmillan.

Hofäcker, D., & Naumann, E. (2015). The emerging trend of work and retirement in Germany: Increasing social inequality? *Zeitschrift für Gerontologie und Geriatrie, 48*(5), 473–479. https://doi.org/10.1007/s00391-014-0669-y

Hyde, M., Cheshire-Allen, M., Damman, M., Platts, L., Pritchard, K., & Reed, C. (2018). *The experience of the transition to retirement: Rapid evidence review*. London, England: Centre for Ageing Better.

James, J., & Pitt-Catsouphes, M. (2016). Change in the meaning and experience of work in later life: Introduction to the special issue. *Work, Ageing and Retirement, 2*(3), 281–285. https://doi.org/10.1093/workar/waw020

Kalleberg, A. L. (2018). *Precarious lives: Job insecurity and well-being in rich democracies*. Cambridge, UK: Polity Press.

Kendig, H., & Nazroo, J. (2016). Life course influences in later life: Comparative perspectives. *Journal of Population Ageing, 9*(1–2), 1–8. https://doi.org/10.1007/s12062-015-9138-7

Koenig, G., Trawinski, L., & Rix, S. (2015). *The long road back: Struggling to find work after unemployment* (American Association of retired persons). Washington, DC: Public Policy Institute.

Kohli, M., Rein, M., Guillemard, A.-M., & van Gunsteren, H. (1991). *Time for retirement: Comparative studies of early exit from the labor force*. Cambridge, UK: Cambridge University Press.

Kojola, E., & Moen, P. (2016). No more lock-step retirement: Boomers shifting meanings of work and retirement. *Journal of Aging Studies, 36*, 59–70. https://doi.org/10.1016/j.jaging.2015.12.003

König, S., Hess, M., & Hofäcker, D. (2016). Trends and determinants of retirement transition in Europe, the USA and Japan: A comparative overview. In D. Hofäcker, M. Hess, & M. S. König (Eds.), *Delaying retirement: Progress and challenges of active ageing in Europe, the United States and Europe* (pp. 25–31). London, England: Palgrave Macmillan.

Kröger, T., & Bagnato, A. (2018). Care for older people in early twenty-first-century Europe: Dimensions and directions of change. In F. Martinelli, A. Anttonen, & M. Mätzke (Eds.), *Social services disrupted: Changes, challenges and policy implications for Europe in times austerity* (pp. 201–218). Cheltenham, UK: Edward Elgar.

Laczko, F., & Phillipson, C. (1991). *Changing work and retirement: Social policy and the older worker*. Milton Keynes, UK: Open University Press.

Lain, D. (2016). *Reconstructing retirement: Work and welfare in the USA*. Bristol, UK: Policy Press.

Lain, D., Airey, L., Loretto, W., & Vickerstaff, S. (2019). Understanding older work precarity: The intersecting domains of jobs, households and the welfare state. *Ageing & Society, 39*(10), 2219–2242. https://doi.org/10.1017/S0144686X18001253

Lain, D., & Phillipson, C. (2019). Extended working lives and the rediscovery of the 'disadvantaged' older worker. *Generations: Journal of the American Society on Aging, 43*, 71–77.

Lewis, J. (2006). Work/Family reconciliation, equal opportunities and social policy: The interpretation of policy trajectories at the EU level and the meaning of gender equality. *Journal of European Public Policy, 13*(3), 76–104. https://doi.org/10.1080/13501760600560490

Loretto, W., & Vickerstaff, S. (2015). Gender, age and flexible working in later life. *Work, Employment & Society, 29*(2), 233–249. https://doi.org/10.1177/0950017014545267

Macnicol, J. (2015). *Neoliberalising old age*. Cambridge, UK: Cambridge University Press.

McDonald, L., & Donahue, P. (2011). Retirement lost. *Canadian Journal on Aging, 30*, 401–422. https://doi.org/10.1017/S0714980811000298

Nì Léime, Á., & Loretto, W. (2017). Gender perspectives on working life policies. In Á. Nì Léime, D. Street, S. Vickerstaff, C. Krekula, & W. Loretto (Eds.), *Gender, ageing and extended working life: Cross-national perspectives* (pp. 53–76). Bristol, UK: Policy Press.

Nì Léime, Á., & Ogg, J. (2019). Gender impacts of extended working life on the health and economic well-being of older workers. *Ageing & Society, 39*(10), 2163–2170. https://doi.org/10.1017/S0144686X18001800

Office for National Statistics. (2019a). *Living longer: Caring in working life*. London, England: Author.

Office for National Statistics. (2019b). *The probability of automation in England: 2011 and 2017*. London, England: Author.

Organisation of Economic Cooperation and Development. (2006). *Live longer, work longer*. Paris, France: Author.

Organisation of Economic Cooperation and Development. (2017). *Pensions at a glance 2017*. Paris, France: Author.

Organisation of Economic Cooperation and Development. (2019a). *The future of work: Employment outlook 2019*. Paris, France: Author.

Organisation of Economic Cooperation and Development. (2019b). *Working better with age*. Paris, France: Author.

Phillipson, C. (1981). Pre-retirement education: The British and American experience. *Ageing & Society*, *1*(3), 393–413.

Phillipson, C. (2013). *Ageing*. Cambridge, UK: Polity Press.

Phillipson, C. (2019). "Fuller" or "extended" working lives: Critical perspectives on changing transitions from work to retirement. *Ageing & Society*, *39*(3), 629–650. https://doi.org/10.1017/S0144686X18000016

Rinklake, A., & Buchholz, S. (2011). Increasing inequalities in Germany: Older people's employment lives and income conditions since the mid-1980s. In H.-P. Blossfeld, S. Buchholz, & K. Kurz (Eds.), *Ageing, globalization and the labour market: Comparing late working life and retirement in modern societies* (pp. 5–64). Cheltenham, UK: Edward Elgar.

Rutledge, M., Wettstein, G., & King, S. (2019). Will more workers have non-traditional jobs as globalization and automation spread?*(Working paper 2019–2010)*. Boston, MA: Center for Retirement Research at Boston College.

Savage, M. (2015). *Social class in the 21st century*. London, England: Pelican Books.

Sennett, R., & Cobb, J. (1977). *The hidden injuries of class*. Cambridge, UK: Cambridge University Press.

Smeaton, D., & White, M. (2016). The growing discontents of older British employees: Extended working life at risk from quality of working life. *Social Policy & Society*, *15*(3), 369–385. https://doi.org/10.1017/S1474746415000366

Srnicek, N., & Williams, A. (2015). *Inventing the future: Postcapitalism and a world without work*. London, England: Verso Books.

Standing, G. (2011). *The precariat: The new dangerous class*. London, England: Bloomsbury.

Standing, G. (2014). *A precariat charter: From denizens to citizens*. London, England: Bloomsbury.

Street, D. (2017). The empirical landscape of extending working lives. In A. Léime, D. Street, S. Vickerstaff, C. Krekula, & W. Loretto (Eds.), *Gender, ageing and extended working life: Cross-national perspectives* (pp. 193–216). Bristol, UK: Policy Press.

Street, D., & Tompkins, J. (2018). Is 70 the new 60? Extending American women's and men's working lives. In Á. Nì Léime, D. Street, S. Vickerstaff, C. Krekula, & W. Loretto (Eds.), *Gender, ageing and extended working life: Cross-national perspectives* (pp. 3–27). Bristol, UK: Policy Press.

Taylor, P. (2019). Working longer may be good public policy, but it is not necessarily good for older people. *Journal of Aging & Social Policy*, *31*(2), 99–105. https://doi.org/10.1080/08959420.2019.1576487

Vickerstaff, S. (2006). Entering the retirement zone: How much choice do individuals have. *Social Policy & Society*, 5, 507–519. https://doi.org/10.1017/S147474640 6003265

Vickerstaff, S. (2015). Retirement. Evolution, revolution or retrenchment. In J. Twigg & W. Martin (Eds.), *Routledge handbook of cultural gerontology* (pp. 297–304). London, England: Routledge.

Vickerstaff, S., & Cox, J. (2005). Retirement and risk: The individualisation of retirement experiences. *Sociological Review*, 53(1), 77–95. https://doi.org/10.1111/j.1467-954X.2005.00504.x

Vickerstaff, S., Street, D., Nì Léime, Á., & Krekula, C. (2017). Gendered and extended work: Research and policy needs for work in later life. In Á. Nì Léime, D. Street, S. Vickerstaff, C. Krekula, & W. Loretto (Eds.), *Gender, ageing and extended working life: Cross-national perspectives* (pp. 219–242). Bristol, UK: Policy Press.

Wainwright, D., Crawford, J., Loretto, W., Phillipson, C., Robinson, M., Shepherd, S., & Weyman, A. (2019). Extending working life and the management of change. Is the workplace ready for the older worker? *Ageing & Society*, 39(11), 2397–2419. https://doi.org/10.1017/S0144686X18000569

Wall, K., & Abiom, S. (2016). Gender in ageing Portugal: Following the lives of men and women. Population ageing from a life course perspective. K. Komp & S. Johansson (Eds.), *Critical and international approaches* (pp. 65–83). Bristol, UK: Policy Press.

Wang, M., Olson, D. A., & Schultz, K. S. (2013). *Mid and late career issues: An integrative perspective*. New York, NY: Routledge.

Wang, M., & Schultz, K. S. (2010). Employee retirement: A review and recommendations for future investigation. *Journal of Management*, 36, 172–206. https://doi.org/10.1037/a0022414

Weller, C. (2016). *Retirement on the rocks*. London, England: Palgrave Macmillan.

Zhu, R., & He, X. (2015). How does women's life satisfaction respond to retirement? A two stage analysis. *Economic Letters*, 137, 118–122. https://doi.org/10.1016/j.econlet.2015.11.002

CHAPTER 2

Neoliberalism and the Future of Retirement Security

Larry Polivka

ABSTRACT

The main questions addressed in this article are: (a) what is the economic status of current retirees and the projected status of future retirees; (b) how does the status of current and future retirees vary by race, gender, socioeconomic status, and age; (c) what are the major forces responsible for trends in retirement security over the last 40 years and the future; and (d) what policy changes are most needed to ensure adequate retirement income and healthcare. The article draws on the available literature to show that while most retirees are economically secure, a growing number, especially among minority and women retirees, are increasingly at risk of being worse off in retirement than they were when working. The main reason for the erosion of retirement security is the shift from defined benefit (DB) private pension plans with guaranteed benefits to defined contribution (DC) plans with benefits determined by the investment decisions of workers and the performance of equities markets. DC plans on the whole do not provide benefits comparable to those historically provided by DB plans. The second major reason for declining retirement security is rising health and long-term care costs that are outstripping the incomes of most retirees. These trends are discussed in the context of neoliberal capitalism and the rise of the corporate or what Wolfgang Streeck calls the Consolidation State. The final section describes policy initiatives needed to end the erosion of retirement security which is largely dependent on a qualitative strengthening of Social Security and major improvements in Medicare.

INTRODUCTION

The financial status of current and future retirees has been a topic of debate and a considerable body of research for several years. The debate has become more urgent since the financial collapse in 2008, the Great Recession that occurred from 2008 until 2010, and the historically slow recovery that followed. Most analysts of retirement security, as shown in the first section of this chapter, tend to conclude that current retirees are on the whole doing reasonably well in maintaining their preretirement standard of living. At the same time, however, a substantial percentage of retirees with low income work careers, which includes many minority and women retirees, are facing financial shortfalls that put them at greater risk of declining incomes and even impoverishment in retirement.

These concerns are based on research into current trends in retirement savings and other indicators of financial security in retirement. The first section of this chapter summarizes the latest research on the financial status of current retirees and the major reasons for the erosion in financial security for many future retirees.

The second section of the chapter discusses the origins of these growing threats to retirement security in the neoliberal political economy that displaced the system of managed welfare state capitalism in the late 1970s and early 1980s. This analysis draws on the theory of the Hayekian Consolidation State developed by the German sociologist Wolfgang Streeck (2014, 2016). Streeck's theory of the role of the state as it has evolved over the last 40 years provides a coherent framework for critiquing neoliberalism as it directly impacts current workers and future retirees through state policies and programs that threaten to erode financial security for future retirees.

The final section of the chapter discusses policy initiatives needed to reverse the negative effects of neoliberalism in both the public and private sectors on workers and their prospects for a financially secure retirement.

ECONOMIC SECURITY OF CURRENT AND FUTURE RETIREES

The growth of inequality in the United States over the last 40 years is reflected in the inequality of retirement savings among working age Americans, most of whom have no retirement savings. The total value of 401(k) and Individual Retirement Accounts (IRAs) reached $16.9 trillion in 2017, but this retirement savings wealth is concentrated in the top income quartile, especially the top

10% of earners. Only 4% of working age Americans have any retirement account assets. These workers have three times the annual income of those without retirement account assets. Even among workers who hold retirement accounts, the average account holder has an account balance of only $40,000. Among those workers age 55 to 64 with retirement accounts, 68% have account balances equal to less than one time their annual incomes, which is far below the 7 to 10 times annual income that most experts in retirement finances recommend to ensure economic security in retirement (Bond & Rhee, 2019).

Thirty-five percent of workers age 55 to 64 have no private retirement account savings or DB pension coverage from a current or past job, which is the main reason the median retirement account balance of older workers (55–64) is only $15,000. Half of all low-income older workers (less than $40,000 annually) have neither retirement savings nor a DB pension. Even among workers with retirement accounts, the savings is extremely low with a median account balance of only $92,000. For this group of workers, more than half are projected to be able to draw retirement income of *less than 15% of their preretirement income* (Brown, Saad-Lessler, & Oakley, 2018; Ghilarducci, Papadopoulos, & Webb, 2017).

This rather bleak perspective on private sources of retirement security for current American workers does not change qualitatively by counting individual net worth. Over 76% of American workers fail to achieve conservative retirement savings goals. Growing income and wealth inequality over the last 50 years has played a major role in this divergence in retirement savings and the future of retirement security (Brown et al., 2018; Ghilarducci et al., 2017).

A recent analysis found that financial asset inequality has increased among Baby Boomers since 2004, as the wealthiest 5% of them saw their share of financial assets grow from 52% in 2014 to 60% in 2016, from 68% to 75% among the top 10% wealthiest and from 86% to 91% among the top 25% wealthiest. In other words, the wealthiest quartile of Baby Boomers own more than 90% of the financial assets for its cohort. On the other hand, the percentage of assets owned by the bottom 50% decreased from a meager 3% to 2% between 2004 and 2016 (Bond & Rhee, 2019). This growing asset inequality shows no sign of abating as these levels of asset concentrations have been reached among Millennials and Generation X at younger ages than the Boomer generation. This trend is especially evident among Millennials, among whom the wealthiest quartile owned 87% of their cohort's financial assets in 2016, which is two decades younger than when the Boomers hit that mark (Brown, 2018). These trends reflect the growth of income and wealth inequality since the 1970s and tax incentives for retirement savings and employer-based retirement plans that advantage more affluent workers (Miller, 2019).

According to a 2019 report from the Economic Policy Institute (Morrissey 2019b), the growing inequality in retirement security reflects a broken retirement system (see Figure 2.1).

The shift from traditional defined benefit (DB) pensions to 401(k)-style defined contribution (DC) plans was an experiment that failed, widening the gap between retirement haves and have-nots. Families at the 90th percentile in the savings distribution had $320,000 or more saved in retirement accounts in 2016, more than triple what they had in 1989. Meanwhile, the median family (at the 50th percentile) had only $7,800 in 2016, and has lost ground since the Great Recession. (Morrissey, 2019a)

Roughly half of private-sector workers do not participate in employer retirement plans. In most cases because they have no choice. Though many people will participate in employer-based plans at some point in their lives, spotty contributions to DC plans—combined with high fees and other leakages from these plans—mean that half of U.S. households are likely to see a sharp decline

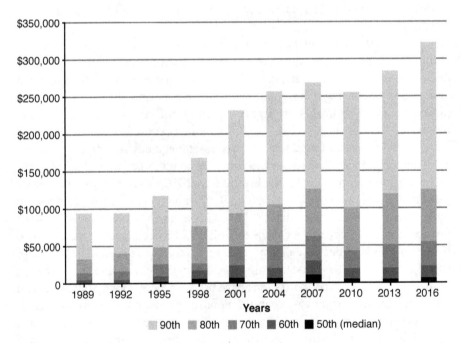

FIGURE 2.1 Retirement account savings of families age 32 to 61 by savings percentile, 1989 to 2016 (2016 dollars).
Source. Data from Morrissey, M. (2019a). *The state of American retirement savings—How the shift to 401(k)s has increased gaps in retirement preparedness based on income, race, ethnicity, education, and marital status.* Economic Policy Institute.

in their standard of living after retiring, especially since Social Security benefits have also been cut back. (Morrissey, 2019a; Munnell, Hou, & Sanzenbacher, 2018a)

The growing reliance on personal retirement accounts is a major reason retirement inequality has increased since the 1980s. The 401(k) system has failed the three basic tests that determine the effectiveness of any retirement programs. According to Morrissey (2019a):

> The 401(k) system fails on all three counts. Too little money is going into 401(k) plans, mainly because many workers do not have the option to participate in a plan at work or earn too little. And money leaks out before retirement in the form of high fees, loans, and withdrawals. Finally, these plans do not pool risk, so contributions need to be much higher to ensure that participants do not outlive their savings. (Morrissey, 2019a)

The erosion of retirement security in the United States is a function of several variables that have not worked to the advantage of most Americans for almost four decades including stagnant wages, increasing debt, the decline of DB pension plans and increasing healthcare costs. These trends have increased the level of financial risk likely to confront retirees in the future, especially those already facing greater financial risks in retirement. Minorities, women and younger workers have much less in retirement wealth assets and as a result are at substantially greater risk of falling short financially in retirement.

African Americans and Hispanics have only a fraction of the median net wealth of White Americans (Munnell, Hou, & Sanzenbacher, 2018b). The ratio of median net wealth of White Americans to African Americans has increased from 4.7 in 2007 to 7.2 in 2016, and for Hispanics the ratio increased from 3.1 to 5.4. These changes reflect the disproportionate impact of the Great Recession and the loss of housing values and wealth, including home foreclosures, on minority families and individuals (Brown & Oakley, 2018; Hou & Sanzenbacher, 2019; Johnson, Mudrazija, & Wang, 2016; Munnell et al., 2018b; Rhee, 2013a). The ratios for household earnings is much less though still significant at 1.8 for both African Americans and Hispanic Americans in 2016. The fact that minorities have so much less net wealth is largely a result of the highly discriminatory, even predatory practices by the real estate and financial services industries toward minority communities in the sale and rental of housing (Taylor, 2019). These practices have made it historically difficult for minorities to achieve housing-based wealth, which is the principal source of accumulated wealth for working and middle-class families. Minorities are also disproportionately the target of exploitative practices in the housing rental markets virtually everywhere in the United States (Taylor, 2019).

In an analysis that focuses more narrowly on comparative retirement wealth, Hou and Sanzenbacher (2019) found that though the gap between White and non-White households is not as great as the gap in total household wealth it is still very substantial as shown in Figure 2.2.

These data clearly indicate the overriding importance of Social Security benefits in compensating for the absence of other sources of retirement wealth which are far more available to Whites than minorities. Without Social Security and to a lesser, but very significant, extent Medicare and Medicaid, African Americans, and Hispanics would have far less retirement wealth than Whites.

In her study of racial disparities in retirement security in the United States, Rhee (2013b) found that 62%and 68% of African American and Hispanic working age households do not own retirement accounts compared to 37% of White households and that these gaps persist across age groups. She also reports that three out of four African American households and four out of five Hispanic working-age households have less than $10,000 in retirement savings compared

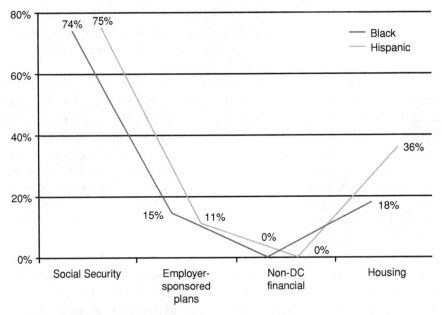

FIGURE 2.2 Wealth for Black and Hispanic households in the middle quintile relative to White households, 2016.
Note. Cases where the typical minority household has negative housing or non-DC financial wealth appear as 0.
Source. Data from Hou, W., & Sanzenbacher, G. T. (2019). *Measuring racial/ethical inequality in retirement wealth.* 21st Annual SSA Research Consortium Meeting, August 1 & 2, 2019.

to 50% of White households. A study by Unidos USA and the National Institute on Retirement Security found that among Hispanic households with retirement savings, they have only one third the average savings of White households and less than 1% of Hispanic households have savings equal to or greater than their annual income (Brown & Oakley, 2018).

A significant part of these differences in retirement savings can be accounted for by differences in educational attainment. As Hispanics continue to increase their attainment levels over the next several years, their ages and savings are likely to grow and bolster their retirement savings, though a substantial gap with White households are also likely to remain (Johnson et al., 2016).

Although the gaps in retirement savings between women and men are not as great as those along racial and ethnic lines, they are still very substantial putting more women at greater risk than men of experiencing retirement income shortfalls. A study by Brown, Rhee, Saad-Lessler, and Oakley (2016) found that among women with retirement savings the median value in women's Defined Contribution (DC) accounts was onethird less than the median amount in the accounts held by men and that the median household incomes of women age 65 plus was 26% less than income for men. Women who are widowed, divorced, and over age 70 rely on Social Security benefits for most of their income. Women age 65 and older are 80% more likely than men to be living in poverty and women age 75 to 79 are three times as likely as men to be impoverished. Even as more women enter retirement with greater savings generated by rising incomes during their working years, these gaps, including a substantially greater rate of impoverishment, are likely to persist well into the future.

Retirement security varies by age group with younger cohorts, especially Millennials, already experiencing worrisome shortfalls in retirement savings. A recent study by Brown (2018) found that 66.8% of working Millennials have no retirement savings and that according to a consensus of financial experts, only 5% of them are saving at sufficient levels for a financially secure retirement. One reason for these shortfalls is that only half of working Millennials whose employers offer a retirement plan actually participate in them. Participation rates vary considerably by race/ethnicity and gender with only about 20% of Hispanic Millennials participating in available employer plans compared to 41.4% of Asian male Millennials and 40.3% of Millennial White women (Brown, 2018). These data indicate that younger workers may be at greater financial risk in retirement than current retirees and even more dependent on Social Security and other public programs, including Medicare and Medicaid, than Boomer and Generation X retirees.

The threats to retirement security facing younger works are being generated by several economic, social, and demographic trends that have emerged over the last several decades, including the precipitous decline of employer sponsored DB pension plans, the increases in Social Security's full retirement age from 65 to 67, stagnating employment and median wages for men, which reduce retirement benefits and the capacity of workers to save, and a sharp decline in median household wealth after 2007 (Johnson, Smith, Cosic, & Wang, 2017). These trends are offset to some extent by the greater extent to which Generation X and Millennial women have worked in their 20s and 30s and earned higher incomes than women in previous cohorts. Further, a substantially higher percentage of Millennial men and women have 4-year college degrees than earlier cohorts. Even with these positive trends, however, a higher proportion of Generation X and Millennials than Boomers will experience a decline in their living standards after retirement due to the more negative trends like the sharp decline in workers participating in DB plans and the falling Social Security income replacement rate (Brown, 2018).

These are two of the major reasons the National Retirement Risk Index (NRRI) developed by the Center for Retirement Research (CRR) shows that the replacement rate will fall over the next several decades with an especially detrimental impact on Millennials in retirement (Munnell et al., 2018a).

The percentage of future retirees whose standard of living may be adversely affected by retirement income shortfalls could be even higher than currently projected by the NRRI model, depending on the financial risks they experience during retirement. The most critical risk is likely to be rising out-of-pocket medical expenses, especially for those over age 80, which is projected to be a rising percentage of future retirees. In fact, the 85+ population is the fastest growing part of the U.S. population and is expected to remain so for several more decades. A study by McInerney, Rutledge, and King (2017) found that the 75+ population paid about 20% of their income to cover out-of-pocket medical expenses. A study by Jones, De Nardi, French, McGee, and Kirschner (2018) estimates that the average age 70+ household will pay about $100,000 in total for out-of-pocket medical expenses and the top 5% of spenders will pay almost $300,000 in out-of-pocket costs. High out-of-pocket medical care expenses are not the only source of financial risk facing retirees as they grow older. A 2019 CRR report (Rutledge & Sanzenbacher, 2019) concludes that:

> The takeaway from these studies seems similar to those on out-of-pocket expenses: the financial threat posed by cognitive decline is smaller today than it may be in the future. So far, cognitive decline has affected the finances of some individuals, but far from a majority. The mitigating factor seems to be having a source of help, and most people have it. However, in the future, having such assistance will be more important, as less income comes from Social Security and traditional pensions and more comes in a lump sum that is more

vulnerable to fraud. In addition, tomorrow's retirees will have fewer children to support them than their parents did, and children are a primary source of financial management assistance. (Rutledge & Sanzenbacher, 2019)

Although consumer debt is not as great a threat to retirement security as rising out-of-pocket healthcare costs, the shift from DB pensions to DC plans and the declining wage replacement capacity of Social Security, it is important to recognize that consumer debt in the 65+ population rose by 250% between 2001 and 2016 and could become a major financial risk for retirees within a few years (National Council on Aging [NCOA], 2018). This risk could be made more serious by increasing numbers of workers entering retirement carrying high debt loads, especially mortgage, credit card, and student debt (Sass, 2018).

The future of retirement security is shaped by several factors, including the wage stagnation that has occurred over the last several decades, especially for workers in middle and lower income groups, growing inequality, which is a result of wage stagnation for most workers and the huge growth in income and wealth gains of the top 1 to 10%, and the steady growth of the costs of housing, education, and healthcare. The medical cost burden for the 65 and older population is projected to increase steadily over time if costs grow at the intermediate rate projected by the Medicare Trustees in 2009 (Johnson & Mommaerts, 2010). According to the authors' projection model results, median out-of-pocket costs will more than double in constant 2008 dollars, from $2,600 in 2010 to about $6,200 in 2040 and 10% of the 65+ population will spend more than $14,000 out-of-pocket in 2040. Although median household income for the age 65+ population is projected to grow during this period, from $26,800 in 2010 to $34,600 by 2040, it is a much slower rate of growth than is projected for healthcare costs.

The growing gap between increases in medical care costs and retirement income will cause the percentage of income spent on medical care to grow from 10% at the median in 2010 to 19% in 2040. The percentage spending more than 20% of their income on medical care will increase from 18% in 2010 to 35% in 2035 and 45% by 2040. They also project that if employers eliminate all retiree health benefits, a trend already well underway, by 2040, the percentage spending over 20% will grow to 52%. If these projections prove to be accurate medical care spending will consume 60% of the real growth in retiree incomes between 2010 and 2040.

These projected increases in medical costs will create especially difficult circumstances for lower income retirees. The median out-of-pocket spending for healthcare among the 65+ population with annual incomes in the bottom 20%

will grow from 21% in 2010 to 39% by 2040, while the increase for those in the top 20% will be only 3%, from 5% to 8%. About 70% of the bottom 40% are projected to spend more than 20% of their income on healthcare.

It should be noted that these projections are based on future healthcare spending that the Medicare Trustees project will be significantly lower than during the period from 1970 to 2005. Healthcare costs have in fact been lower during the 2010 to 2018 period than from 1970 to 2005 and consistent so far with the 2010 Medicare Trustees projections.

These projections and the other research findings described in this section indicate that the standard of living of most future retirees will depend very substantially on either increasing retiree incomes, containing increases on healthcare costs, both medical and long-term costs, or both. Either approach to protecting the standard of living of future retirees would require major changes in the U.S. economy and public policy agenda, both of which have been dominated by neoliberal priorities such as relatively low taxes on high incomes and wealth, austerity focused public budgets at the federal and state levels, deregulation of business practices, privatization of public programs and other measures designed to shrink governments, unleash markets, and return to greater reliance on individual responsibility for economic security.

NEOLIBERAL CAPITALISM AND RETIREMENT SECURITY

The U.S. political economy as well as those of several European countries have undergone profound changes over the last 40 years. The state guided (managed) welfare state capitalism that emerged from the New Deal state intervention oriented policies of the Roosevelt Administration and state managed war economy of 1941 to 1946 generated what is often called the Golden Age of American Capitalism. This description of the period from 1946 until about 1975 is based on the unprecedented growth of the economy during this period and the extent to which the working class was able to share in the growth (Stein, 2010). Many working class households were able to join the middle class which grew more during this period than in any other period either before 1945 or after 1975. This broad prosperity was generated by several factors including the social programs that were created during the New Deal (Social Security, strong financial regulation, support for the rights of labor in disputes with management, the higher education GI bill, etc.) and early postwar period (Harvey, 2007). The emergence of the United States as the major power in the global economy at the end of World War II was critically important to the high level economic growth during this period. Economic growth alone, however, would not have been sufficient to ensure the kind of uniquely broad prosperity Americans experienced from 1945 to 1975. Keynesian policies of demand stimulation that were adopted during this period could have been implemented in multiple ways, but the fact that they often took the form of funding for social programs like Social Security, employment support and later, Great Society programs like Medicare and Medicaid that were redistributive in nature was essential to ensuring shared prosperity (Polivka, 2012).

The third critical factor in addition to the comparative strength and advantage of the United States in the postwar global economy and the socially oriented Keynesian stimulation policies was the emergence of worker power as union membership growth gave labor the kind of leverage in negotiations with management that led to agreements ensuring increases in wages and benefits (health insurance and pensions) that workers had never been able to achieve before. These private sector benefits, along with Social Security, Medicare and Medicaid constitute the infrastructure for retirement security in the United States. This unprecedented labor strength made it possible for workers to equitably share in the productivity gains that were comparatively high and steady, year to year, throughout the 1945 to 1975 period (Kuttner, 2008).

Since the late 1970s, however, gains in productivity, which slowed substantially after 1980, have gone almost entirely to corporate shareholders and management. This shift in the flow of productivity gains is a major source of the growth in inequality since 1980. It is also one of the first indicators of the great transformation in the United States that began in the mid-1970s and came to full fruition during the Reagan Administration (Kuttner, 2008).

The shift from the state guided welfare state capitalism of the postwar period to what is commonly called neoliberal pro-corporate capitalism was largely a result of the inability of Keynesian policies to resolve the high inflation and slow growth (stagnation) challenges that emerged with the recession in 1974 to 1975 and the APEC oil embargos that drove energy costs to unprecedented levels in 1973 and again at the end of the 1970s (Stein, 2010). An organized corporate effort was launched during that same period to reduce the power of labor unions in wage and benefits negotiations and the role of the state in shaping fiscal and regulatory policies opposed by the business sector (Phillips-Fein, 2009). These fiscal policies included funding for New Deal and Great Society social programs and the use of federal taxes to redistribute money from the wealthy to working and middle-class households.

The retirement security system that was constructed in the postwar period included the development in the private sector of often relatively generous DB-pension plans and retiree health insurance plans and public sector programs from Social Security, which was established during the New Deal to the Medicare and Medicaid programs of the Great Society period in the mid-1960s. This public–private infrastructure for retirement security provided American retirees with unprecedented levels of economic and healthcare security and led to what has been referred to as the Golden Age of Retirement (Hacker, 2002).

As described, however, in the previous sections the private sector retirement benefits began to change in the late 1970s and early 1980s with the move to DC pensions among companies offering a pension plan. Companies also began dropping their retiree health insurance programs and by 2019 fewer than 30% of all companies made such plans available. These changes in retiree benefits were largely the result of shifts in corporate strategies in the 1970s from support for the managed welfare state model of postwar capitalism to a neoliberal model featuring a more antagonistic relationship with labor unions and greater opposition to increasing employee pay and benefits and an aggressive strategy for moving government policy in a pro-corporate direction. These initiatives have largely succeeded in the development of more pro-corporate political and economic environments where the power of labor unions has been dramatically diminished along with employee wages and retirement benefits (Stein, 2010).

The success of corporate interests in rolling back the gains of employees in wages and retiree benefits by taking full advantage of globalization and the growing capacity of corporations to move jobs to lower wage countries and a rejectionist approach to union wage and benefit demands has not been matched yet by similar rollbacks in the public sector retirement programs. This does not mean, however, that corporate interests have not made substantial progress in moving the policy agendas of the federal and several state governments away from the progressive priorities of the managed capitalism period when the U.S. retirement security system was developed to far more pro-corporate priorities across a wide range of policy domains from taxation to healthcare to regulatory policy (Lorey, 2015; Polivka, 2012). This shift in policy priorities is often referred to as the emergence of the neoliberal state, or what the sociologist Wolfgang Streeck refers to as the Hayekian Consolidation State (Streeck, 2014).

The future of retirement security depends increasingly on the survival and strengthening of the two pillars of the public retirement systems, Social Security and Medicare, that were implemented during the New Deal and Great Society periods. Neoliberal proposals to privatize Social Security would, in effect, make the program as risky as private pensions have become with the shift from DB pension plans to DC plans over the last 35 years.

In fact, it is becoming increasingly apparent that Social Security and Medicare are likely to be even more important for the economic security of future retirees than they are for current retirees, especially women, minorities, and lower income workers regardless of gender or race. The increasing importance of both Social Security, Medicare, and Medicaid, which is the principal source of funding for long-term care in the United States, not only makes the preservation of these programs essential, it also points to the need to improve them by increasing benefit levels and reducing out-of-pocket costs for medical and long-term care.

The relentless growth, however, of deficits in the federal budget and the cumulative debt, which now exceeds $23 trillion, and the continuing dominance of the neoliberal political economy and public policy agenda will keep the preservation, much less improvement, of Social Security, Medicare, and Medicaid at risk for the foreseeable future. The survival of neoliberalism in the wake of the financial collapse and Great Recession is testament to how deeply embedded neoliberalism has become in the domestic and global economies and in the structures of the state (Streeck, 2016). Wolfgang Streeck's concept of the Consolidation State offers some insight into why neoliberalism has proven to be so enduring over the last decade as an elite consensus project and why it constitutes such a serious threat to the future of retirement security.

According to Streeck, the Austrian economist and social theorist Frederick Hayek was less an apostle for free markets unregulated by governments than he was an advocate for corporate interests and power. Hayek's major concern was to protect the corporate sector from state interference in the economy whether such interference took the form of Keynesian policies to stimulate growth through increases in public spending or more intrusive socialist interventions including nationalization of whole industries. In addition however, Streeck's analysis of Hayek's thought shows that Hayek supported an active role for the state in shoring up and protecting the corporate sector through regulations designed to help large corporations pursue monopoly control of markets and legislation that protects capital and corporate power from the democratic interests of the public (Streeck, 2014).

The Consolidation State serves its Hayekian mission by protecting corporate interests from regulations designed to limit the growth of monopoly power and fraudulent corporate practices, especially in the financial sector, and from public programs like Social Security and Medicare and taxes on high incomes and wealth to pay for them. On the other hand, the Hayekian state is designed to protect corporate interests by foregoing antitrust actions against monopolies, imposing austerity budgets that keep tax rates on the wealthy low but high enough on the nonwealthy to preserve the capacity of the state to pay for bailouts and pay for enough of the public debt to keep interest rates on the debt from becoming too high (Streeck, 2016).

All of the wealth-preserving and enhancing functions of the Consolidation State are growing threats to the economic security of future retirees who will depend on programs such as Social Security, Medicare and Medicaid to meet their financial and healthcare needs. The Consolidation State is, in short, a powerful vehicle for putting older persons at increasing risk of a precarious retirement (Estes, 2014).

The concept of the Consolidation State or advanced corporate state, is clearly relevant to the neoliberal trends in the U.S. healthcare system that threaten the future of retirement security. As the healthcare system has grown over the last three decades, corporate health firms, mainly large insurance companies, have gained increasing control of the publicly funded healthcare programs through contracts with federal and state governments. Private insurance companies now administer plans that cover over one third of all Medicare beneficiaries through Medicare Advantage (MA) managed care plans and are on track to control over 50% by 2025 (Gaffney, 2015).

Private insurance companies also control over 75% of Medicaid acute care services in most states and are rapidly taking control of Medicaid long-term care programs in many states. The privatization of Medicaid long-term care programs is removing administrative control of community-based services from nonprofit community-based organizations, such as Area Agencies on Aging, by contracting with largely for-profit insurance companies including United Health Care, Centene, Humana, and Aetna (Polivka & Luo, 2017).

The Affordable Care Act (ACA, or Obamacare) expanded insurance coverage and reduced the uninsured population by about 20 million. The ACA also accelerated the shift from nonprofit community-based and -controlled Medicaid long-term care services to corporate control as a growing number of states opt for managed care contracts with insurance companies. The ACA included incentives for states to contract out more of their Medicaid programs through the Medicaid-Medicare Dual Eligible Demonstration program. The Centers for Medicare & Medicaid (CMS) has also loosened oversight of Medicaid managed care programs as documented in recent monitoring reports from the Government Accountability Office (GAO, 2017).

The rapid growth of corporate participation in the Medicare program through MA is another very important source of the neoliberal, pro-corporate turn in the U.S. healthcare system. The growing corporate role in Medicare is fully consistent with one of the original purposes of the MA program, which was to create a vehicle within Medicare to facilitate the privatization of the program. With over one third of Medicare beneficiaries now enrolled in MA, the leverage exercised over the Medicare program by corporate health firms is very substantial and increasing annually (Geyman, 2017). The extent of this leverage is evident in the fact that CMS has been largely ineffective in its oversight responsibilities; MA plans are still more expensive than regular fee-for-service programs and excessive reimbursement through procedure up-coding (providing more expensive services than the beneficiary actually needed) has become a common practice across plans (Gaffney, 2015).

These trends in the U.S. healthcare system, along with the declining value of private pensions, stagnant wages, and low savings are creating conditions favorable to the extension of employment precarity into an increasingly precarious retirement for future retirees (Standing, 2011).

The increasing privatization of healthcare is part of larger neoliberal austerity initiative at the federal and state levels to contain increases in public budgets through contracts with corporations and reduced oversight through deregulation and meager monitoring so that market competition can presumably increase efficiency and contain costs without reducing access and services. We have little evidence that any of these beneficial outcomes are occurring and substantial evidence that they are not. For example, costs in the MA continue to exceed those in regular Medicare and the HMO-contracted Medicaid programs continue to grow at the same or higher rates as they did when the program was mostly fee-for-service (Polivka & Luo, 2017). We also have evidence that the Medicaid HMO program, especially in the long-term care part of Medicaid, is restricting access to care even as contract costs grow. For example in Florida the wait list for long-term care services is growing by 5 to 10,000 annually since HMOs took control of the Medicaid long-term care program and now exceeds 60,000 persons (Florida Council on Aging, 2020).

A large percentage of the privatized funds are spent to meet profit expectations and cover high administrative costs (10%–15%) which means that funds for healthcare for older beneficiaries of Medicare and Medicaid are under increasing pressure at both the sources of appropriation (austerity) and expenditure (administrative costs and profits). This is a recipe for growth of precarity among the elderly who depend on these programs for meeting virtually all of their health and LTC needs (Polivka, 2020).

These neoliberal trends (austerity and privatization) in the direction of greater precarity in retirement are consistent with Wolfgang Streeck's concept of the Consolidation State (advanced corporate state) in neoliberal political economies in the West. The Consolidation State is designed to serve the interest of capital, especially finance capital, by implementing austerity budgets, maintaining low taxes on high incomes and wealth, prioritizing the financing of state deficits and debts (debt consolidation) and privatizing as many profitable public services and assets as possible.

As the Consolidation State tightens its grip on the entire public sector, the precarity of later life is likely to grow as the already extensive privatization of health and LTC is expanded and the original purpose of these public services is subverted by the pursuit of profits through the massive commodification of the need for care. The growth of the Consolidation State and a neoliberal public policy agenda are creating a glide path toward the extension of precarious employment into a precarious retirement for millions of older people over the next several years.

CONCLUSION

The pro-corporate neoliberal political economy and public policy agenda dominated by privatization, deregulation, low taxes on the wealthy, and austerity budgets have materially diminished the retirement security of working and middle-class income households over the last 40 years. These trends are likely to continue as long as the neoliberal policy agenda remains dominant, ensuring that the economic precarity increasingly experienced by workers since the 1970s will emerge in retirement for growing numbers of future retirees. The implementation of large federal economic stimulus programs such as infrastructure investments, student debt relief, higher federal minimum wages, increased education spending, and other neo-Keynesian economic policies designed to benefit working and middle-class families would help blunt neoliberal attacks on federal retirement entitlement programs and create a favorable political and financial environment for progressive initiatives to rebuild retirement security including the following:

- A dual initiative to strengthen the financial foundation of Social Security by upwardly adjusting or even removing the income cap in the payroll tax, and instituting a gradual increase in the payroll tax (i.e., 2% over 20 years), and to increase benefits, especially for low-income beneficiaries.
- A federally guaranteed and administered, forward-funded secondary pension designed to gradually replace current DC private pensions which have proven to be too risky to be an effective substitute for traditional DB plans.
- An overhaul of the Medicare program, including changes in the 2003 Medicare Modernization Act (MMA) designed to reduce the cost of the MA program; contain prescription drug costs (allow price negotiations); to implement a new Medicare program that would consolidate and impose an annual cap on all out-of-pocket costs (premium, co-payments and deductibles) and create a new Medicare benefit to cover long-term care costs.
- Finally a comprehensive program for strong and equitable economic growth should include specific strategies to raise wages which would allow employees to increase their retirement resources through enhanced savings and asset wealth accumulation.

These progressive alternatives to the neoliberal model of a fully privatized retirement security system are likely to be the issues around which the politics of aging will unfold over the next several years. We should anticipate sustained neoliberal resistance to increasing revenues through higher taxes on the wealthy; preserving and strengthening Social Security, Medicare, and Medicaid, the largest source of public support for long-term care services; restructuring the private pension system; and to containing military expenditures that are needed for other priorities including retirement security. If this resistance is successful, the future of retirement security will continue to deteriorate.

REFERENCES

Bond, T., & Rhee, N. (2019, September). *Financial asset inequality and its implications for retirement security*. Washington, DC: National Institute on Retirement Security.

Brown, J., & Oakley, D. (2018, December). *Latinos' retirement insecurity in the United States*. Washington, DC: National Institute on Retirement Security.

Brown, J. E. (2018, February). *Millennials and retirement: Already falling short*. Washington, DC: National Institute on Retirement Security.

Brown, J. E., Rhee, N., Saad-Lessler, J., & Oakley, D. (2016, March). *Shortchanged in retirement-continuing challenges to women's financial future*. Washington, DC: National Institute on Retirement Security.

Brown, J. E., Saad-Lessler, J., & Oakley, D. (2018, September). *Retirement in America: Out of reach for working Americans*. Washington, DC: National Institute on Retirement Security.

Estes, C. L. (2014). The future of aging services in a neoliberal political economy. *Journal of the American Society on Aging, Generations, 38*(2), 94–100.

Florida Council on Aging. (2020). *2020 Legislative Session. 2020 Advocacy Initiative Brochure*. Retrieved from https://fcoa.starchapter.com/images/other/FINAL_Combined_Brochure_2020.pdf

Gaffney, A. (2015). The neoliberal turn in American health care. *International Journal of Health Services, 45*(1), 33–52.

GAO. (2017). *January 2017 (GAO-1-145) and the August 2017 GAO report to Congress "Medicaid Managed Care: CNS Should Improve Oversight of Access and Quality in States' Long Term Services and Supports Programs."* The GAO 2017 studies support the need for much stronger oversight of the states' Medicaid managed LTC programs with a call for CMS to provide minimum standards for encounter data to be reported by states. Washington, DC.

Geyman, J. (2017). Crisis in U.S. health care: Corporate power still blocks reform. *International Journal of Health Services, 48*(1), 5–27. https://doi.org/10.1177/0020731417729654

Ghilarducci, T., Papadopoulos, M., & Webb, A. (2017). *Inadequate retirement savings for workers nearing retirement*. New York, NY: Schwartz Center for Economic Policy

Analysis and Department of Economics, The New School for Social Research, Policy Note Series.

Hacker, J. S. (2002). *The divided welfare state: The battle over public and private social benefits in the United States.* Cambridge, England: Cambridge University Press.

Harvey, D. (2007). *A brief history of neoliberalism.* Oxford, England: Oxford University Press.

Hou, W., & Sanzenbacher, G. T. (2019, August 1 & 2). *Measuring racial/ethical inequality in retirement wealth.* 21st Annual SSA Research Consortium Meeting. National Press Club, Washington, DC.

Johnson, R. W., & Mommaerts, C. (2010, February). *Will health care costs bankrupt aging boomers?.* Urban Institute. Washington, DC.

Johnson, R. W., Mudrazija, S., & Wang, D. X. (2016, December). *Hispanics' retirement security.* Washington, DC: Urban Institute.

Johnson, R. W., Smith, K. E., Cosic, D., & Wang, C. X. (2017, November). *Retirement prospects for the millennials: What is the early prognosis?* Boston, MA: Center for Retirement Research at Boston College.

Jones, J. B., Nardi, De. M., French, E., McGee, R., & Kirschner, J. (2018). *The lifetime medical spending of retirees* (Working paper 24599). Cambridge, MA: National Bureau of Economic Research.

Kuttner, R. (2008). *The squandering of America—how the failure of our politics undermines our prosperity.* New York, NY: Vintage Books.

Lorey, I. (2015). *State of insecurity: Government of the precarious.* London, England: Verso Books.

McInerney, M. P., Rutledge, M. S., & King, S. E. (2017). *How much does out-of-pocket medical spending eat away at retirement income?* (Working paper 2017–13). Chestnut Hill, MA: Center for Retirement Research at Boston College.

Miller, M. (2019, December). The decade in retirement: Wealthy Americans moved further ahead. *The New York Times.* https://www.nytimes.com/2019/12/14/business/retirement-social-security-recession.html

Morrissey, M. (2019a, December). *The state of American retirement savings—how the shift to 401(k)s has increased gaps in retirement preparedness based on income, race, ethnicity, education, and marital status.* Washington, DC: Economic Policy Institute.

Morrissey, M. (2019b, December). *Steady contributions, affordability, and lifetime income are the building blocks of a retirement system that works for working families—Expanding Social Security is the most important step.* Washington, DC: Economic Policy Institute.

Munnell, A. H., Hou, W., & Sanzenbacher, G. T. (2018a, January). *National Retirement Risk Index shows modest improvement in 2016* (Number 18-1). Boston, MA: Center for Retirement Research at Boston College.

Munnell, A. H., Hou, W., & Sanzenbacher, G. T. (2018b, November). *Trends in retirement security by race/ethnicity* (Number 18-21). Boston, MA: Center for Retirement Research at Boston College.

National Council on Aging. (2018). *Older adults and debt: Trends, trade-offs and tools to help.* Washington, DC: Author.

Phillips-Fein, K. (2009). *Invisible hands: The businessmen's crusade against the new deal*. New York, NY: W. W. Norton.

Polivka, L. (2012). The growing neoliberal threat to the economic security of workers and retirees. *The Gerontologist, 52*(1), 133–144. https://doi.org/10.1093/geront/gnr150

Polivka, L., & Luo, B. (2020). Precarious employment to precarious retirement: Neoliberal health and long-term care in the United States (pp. 191–213). In A. Grenier, C. Phillipson, & R. A. Settersten, Jr., *Precarity and ageing: Understanding insecurity and risk in later life*. Bristol, UK: The Policy Press.

Polivka, L., & Luo, B. (2017). Neoliberal long-term care: From community to corporate control. *The Gerontologist, 59*(2), 222–229. https://doi.org/10.1093/geront/gnx139.

Rhee, N. (2013a, June). *The retirement savings crisis: Is it worse than we think?* Washington, DC: National Institute on Retirement Security.

Rhee, N. (2013b, December). *Race and retirement insecurity in the United States*. Washington, DC: National Institute on Retirement Security.

Rutledge, M. S., & Sanzenbacher, G. T. (2019, January). *What financial risks do retirees face in late life?* (Number 19-1). Boston, MA: Center for Retirement Research at Boston College.

Sass, S. A. (2018, February). *Will the financial fragility of retirees increase?* (Number 18-4). Boston, MA: Center for Retirement Research at Boston College.

Standing, G. (2011). *The precariat: The new dangerous class*. London, England: Bloomsbury.

Stein, J. (2010). *Pivotal decade: How the United States traded factories for finance in the seventies*. New Haven, CT: Yale University Press.

Streeck, W. (2014). *Buying time: The delayed crisis of democratic capitalism*. London, England: Verso.

Streeck, W. (2016). *How will capitalism end*. Brooklyn, NY: Verso.

Taylor, K. (2019). *Race for profit: How banks and the real estate industry undermined black homeownership (justice, power, and politics)*. Chapel Hill, NC: The University of North Carolina Press.

CHAPTER 3

Families in Later Life

A Consequence and Engine of Social Inequalities

Deborah Carr

ABSTRACT

The implications of economic inequality for American families are profound, giving rise to widening race and socioeconomic disparities in key family transitions
including marriage, divorce, cohabitation, childrearing, and family bereavement.
However, little scholarly attention focuses on how these divergences in family
structure shape the health and well-being of older adults, and especially older
women. In this chapter, I propose that family relationships are an important
although overlooked mechanism linking economic inequality to persistent race,
socioeconomic, and gender disparities in late-life well-being. I provide a statistical
snapshot of older adults' families, showing how rates of marriage, divorce, widowhood, and remarriage differ markedly on the basis of gender, socioeconomic
status, and race, with these disparities widening against the backdrop of rising
economic inequality in the late 20th and early 21th centuries. I then describe
how these patterns perpetuate disparities in late-life economic well-being, due
in part to the structure of Social Security benefits which advantage those whose
family lives conformed to the mid-20th century White middle-class "ideal" of
a lifelong marriage between a male breadwinner and female homemaker. I further show how three stressful aspects of family lives — family bereavement, custodial grandparenting, and caregiving — disproportionately befall women, and

© 2020 Springer Publishing Company
http://dx.doi.org/10.1891/0198-8794.40.43

especially low-income and women of color. As such, these family-related stressors exacerbate race, class, and gender-based disparities in health and well-being. I conclude by highlighting social policies that may help to mitigate against these disparities, and provide resources so that Americans of all backgrounds have an opportunity to grow old with dignity.

INTRODUCTION

Levels of economic inequality in the United States have risen dramatically over the past five decades, and in the early 2000s reached their most extreme level since shortly before the Great Depression of the early 1930s (Congressional Budget Office, 2019; Piketty, 2014). Since the late 1960s, the income and wealth levels of the top 5% of earners in the United States have climbed steeply, whereas growth has been much more muted or even flat among those at lower rungs of the economic ladder (Congressional Budget Office, 2019). The implications of economic inequality for American families are profound, giving rise to widening race and socioeconomic disparities in whether and the age at which people make important family transitions including marriage, divorce, cohabitation, childrearing, and even family bereavement (e.g., Gibson-Davis & Percheski, 2018; Lundberg, Pollak & Stearns, 2016; Smock & Schwartz, 2020; Umberson et al., 2017). Researchers and policy makers have documented the powerful consequences of these divergent family structures for the economic, physical, emotional, and cognitive well-being of children born into those families (e.g., Gibson-Davis & Percheski, 2018; Lundberg et al., 2016; Pickett & Wilkinson, 2015). However, scholars have not paid comparable attention to how these divergences in family structure shape the health and well-being of older adults, with their effects intensifying over the life course, and exacting a particularly harsh toll on the well-being of older women.

I propose that family relationships are an important although overlooked mechanism linking economic inequality to persistent race, socioeconomic, and gender disparities in late-life well-being. Family relationships are critical to one's health, wealth, and happiness. Married persons enjoy greater economic stability, better mental health, and longer and healthier lives relative to their counterparts who have never married or whose marriages ended through divorce or spousal death (Carr & Springer, 2010; Carr & Utz, 2020). Yet the family structures conferring the greatest benefits are precisely those entered into and maintained by persons with the greatest social and economic advantages; as such, families are a critical engine driving processes of cumulative advantage and disadvantage over the life course.

This chapter opens with a statistical snapshot of older adults' families, showing how rates of marriage, divorce, widowhood, and remarriage differ markedly on the basis of gender, socioeconomic status, and race, with these disparities widening against the backdrop of rising economic inequality in the late 20th and early 21st centuries. I then describe how these patterns perpetuate disparities in late-life economic well-being, due in part to the structure of Social Security benefits which advantage those whose family lives conformed to the mid-20th century White middle-class "ideal" of a lifelong marriage between a male breadwinner and female homemaker. I further show how three stressful aspects of family life—family bereavement, custodial grandparenting, and caregiving—disproportionately befall women, and especially low-income women and women of color. As such, these family-related stressors exacerbate race, class, and gender-based disparities in health and well-being. I conclude by highlighting social policies that may help to mitigate against these disparities, and provide resources so that Americans of all backgrounds have an opportunity to grow old with dignity.

LATER-LIFE FAMILIES: A STATISTICAL SNAPSHOT

Marriage was a near universal institution in the United States in the mid-20th century, although in recent decades it has become recognized as an institution of racial, economic, and gender privilege (Cherlin, 2010). Whites and persons with higher levels of income and education are more likely than Blacks and financially vulnerable persons to marry and stay married, and are more likely to remarry following marital dissolution (Cohen & Pepin, 2018; Raley, Sweeney, & Wondra, 2015; Shafer & James, 2013). Men are more likely than women to remain married "until death do us part," whereas women are more likely to become widowed. Women also are less likely to remarry following divorce or widowhood (Brown, Lin, Hammersmith & Wright, 2016).

Older men are more likely than older women to be currently married, and this gender gap increases with age. Among adults ages 65 to 74, three quarters of men yet just 58% of women are currently married (U.S. Census, 2015). By ages 85 and older, 59% of men yet just 17% of women are still married. For current cohorts of older adults, this disparity largely reflects the widowhood gap. Wives tend to outlive their husbands, a reality exacerbated by the fact that men tend to marry women 2 to 3 years younger than themselves, on average (England & McClintock, 2009). Race gaps also are pronounced. Blacks are more likely than Whites to be unmarried, whether never married, divorced, or widowed, and the race gap in marriage has widened considerably over the past six decades (Raley et al., 2015). In 2015, 72% of White men ages 65+ were currently married compared to just 54% of Black men. An even more pronounced race gap is evident among women; 44% of White women yet just 23% of Black women ages 65+ are married, a function of Blacks' higher rates of divorce, widowhood, and remaining single for life. While lifelong singlehood is rare among current cohorts of older adults, it is twice as common among Black men and women (8.7% and 9.4%) relative to White men and women (4.4% and 4.1%).

Gender and race gaps in marital status mean that older women and especially women of color are more likely than men to live alone, an established risk factor for many physical and mental health concerns including falls, loneliness, cognitive impairment, and mortality risk (e.g., Painter, Elliott, & Hudson, 2009; Smith & Victor, 2019). Men tend to spend their later years at home, with their wife by their side. Older women, especially women of color, do not have this luxury. Fully 43% of Black women ages 65+ live on their own, compared to just 20% of White men. Conversely, just 24% of older Black women live with a spouse, whereas roughly two thirds of men do. Given the centrality of marriage to older adults' well-being, race and gender gaps in family structure are a powerful mechanism contributing to and exacerbating later-life inequalities (Carr, 2019).

THE IMPACT OF FAMILY STRUCTURE ON LATE-LIFE ECONOMIC SECURITY

Marriage is a critical pathway to economic security, yet getting married and remaining married are benefits that are increasingly out of reach for women, Blacks, and persons of lower socioeconomic status. As such, marriage is a key engine perpetuating and widening economic disparities. Being married brings sustained financial benefits over the life course, whereas ending a marriage entails economic costs, with these decrements particularly severe for women, and especially women of color. Spouses enjoy economies of scale, such that their pooled income and savings go further in covering expenses for shared resources like food, secure housing, and heating bills (Smock, Manning, & Gupta, 1999). For older couples in which both partners are working for pay (or who did work for pay in their preretirement years), two incomes go further than one in covering daily expenses and provide a financial cushion in the event of a health crisis or other emergency (Carr, 2019).

Marriage also has been a main pathway through which current cohorts of older women received health insurance in their preretirement years; for women working in part-time jobs or those not working for pay, their husband's employer was the primary source of health insurance (Angel, Montez, & Angel, 2011). However, the economic benefits of marriage are consistently larger for Whites relative to Black and Latinx persons, a consequence of the higher earnings, better quality jobs, and greater access to benefits like health insurance among Whites (Semyonov, Lewin-Epstein, & Bridges, 2011). These racial gaps in the economic benefits bestowed upon older married women have widened in recent decades, alongside rising levels of income inequality (Manduca, 2018).

Married persons also are spared the direct costs associated with marital dissolution such as legal fees in the case of divorce, and medical and funeral expenditures related to a spouse's death (Fan & Zick, 2006). The latter are especially daunting to Blacks, who are less likely than Whites to have life insurance to help defray costly funeral expenses (Harris & Yelowitz, 2018). Women are particularly vulnerable to dissolution-related declines in their standard of living (Bianchi, 1999) and household income (Leopold, 2018), and increased risks of poverty (Smock et al., 1999) and the loss of homeownership (Dewilde, 2008). Women experience a 25% to 40% drop in their standard of living whereas men experience anywhere from a 10% gain to a 10% drop, where the latter is limited to the small population of men whose wives were the family's primary breadwinner (Tach & Eads, 2015).

Remarriage is an effective pathway to economic stability following marital dissolution, with midlife and older remarried persons faring as well financially as those in first marriages, and both faring significantly better than divorced persons who remain unmarried (Lin, Brown, & Hammersmith, 2017). However, older women are less likely than men to remarry, due to a skewed sex ratio and shortage of potential partners (Wu & Schimmele, 2005), men's tendency to seek out partners younger than themselves (England & McClintock, 2009), and women's desire to maintain their independence and be spared of intensive spousal caregiving (Brown et al., 2016). Black women have particularly low chances of remarriage, given Black men's high rates of mortality. While men are more likely than women to remarry, remarriage—like marriage—is an institution of privilege. White, U.S.-born, and more highly educated men are more likely to remarry, relative to their Black, immigrant, and less educated counterparts (Livingston, Parker, & Ruhal, 2014). This disparity partly reflects the fact that men with more stable careers and higher income are considered more "marriageable" and desirable partners, whereas men with fewer economic advantages are less likely to attract and retain a romantic partner (Sawhill & Venator, 2015; Wilson, 1987).

The Importance of Social Security to Late-Life Financial Security

An important yet overlooked mechanism perpetuating economic disparities in later life is the structure of Social Security benefits, which privileges older adults who have lived what sociologists characterize as a White middle-class life; a long-term marriage between a breadwinner and homemaker. Social Security is a national income security program for older adults, established in the United

States in 1935 and expanded dramatically in the 1970s. The program was originally designed for an era in which most people (especially White middle-class people) married once, remained married for life, maintained a traditional male breadwinner/female homemaker arrangement, and the "breadwinner" had secure and long-term employment (Lin, Brown, & Hammersmith, 2017). When marriages ended, it was typically through widowhood rather than divorce.

Consistent with these early to mid-20th century notions of families, Social Security continues to provide more substantial benefits to married and widowed people, relative to their single and divorced counterparts (Meyer & Herd, 2007). The program design also privileges those who maintained breadwinner/homemaker (rather than dual-earner) arrangements during their preretirement years, and those who married and worked for life rather than for brief or sporadic spells. In practice, these program rules mean that lower-income persons and African Americans are disadvantaged, given their relatively low rates of long-term marriage and high rates of divorce (Raley et al., 2015). Blacks and persons with lower levels of education are further disadvantaged because they are more likely than Whites and highly educated persons to have been in dual-earner couples, requiring two incomes to support their families (Fullerton, 1999).

Social Security is one of the most successful social programs in U.S. history, providing income security to millions of older adults. Without Social Security, 40% of older adults rather than the current 10% would be living beneath the official poverty line (Romig & Sherman, 2016). The program is progressive, meaning that lower-wage earners receive a higher percentage benefit than higher-wage earners. Despite the undeniable success of Social Security, however, more than 4 million older adults in the United States live in poverty today, with women, unmarried persons, and ethnic minorities especially vulnerable because they are largely if not wholly dependent on Social Security for their financial security, and are less likely to have additional income from employer-provided pensions, interest income, or wages. In 2015, one in five Black and Latinx older households subsisted solely on their monthly Social Security checks, compared to just 13% of White households. Social Security accounted for nearly half of older unmarried women's income, compared to just 34% and 29% among unmarried men and older married couples, respectively (U.S. Census Bureau, 2015). Social Security benefits are a necessity for lower-income households. Social Security payments account for more than three quarters of the monthly incomes of lower-income households (at or below 200% of the poverty line), but just 52% and 21% of the household incomes of middle- (between 200% and 400% of the poverty line) and higher-income households (at or above 400% of the poverty line), respectively.

There are several reasons why historically disadvantaged subgroups are so highly dependent on Social Security. Employer-provided pensions, considered the second most important source of retirement income after Social Security, often are out of reach to women, ethnic minorities, and persons with precarious employment. Data from the Current Population Survey show that 57% of wage and salary workers currently work for an employer that sponsors a retirement plan, and just 48% participate in the plan. Workers for larger firms, typically around 100 or more employees, and higher income workers are most likely to receive these benefits. Because Blacks, Latinx, and women are less likely to work for large firms or in higher-wage jobs, they are less likely to have their own employer-provided pension plan. An estimated 62% of Whites, but just 54% of Blacks and Asians, and 38% of Latinx persons have an employer-provided pension (Rhee, 2013). Married women may have access to private pensions through their spouse's job, a benefit that is less often available to women of color and low-income women, who are less likely to marry and stay married, and whose spouses may have poorer quality jobs with fewer benefits (Angel et al., 2011).

Yet even among those who are offered an employer pension, workers who are the most economically secure are best positioned to participate in the plan. Over the past four decades, defined-benefit (DB) pension plans have gradually been replaced by defined-contribution (DC) plans; the latter require that a worker have both the financial wherewithal to save for the future and the investment savvy to do so effectively (Stoltzfus, 2016). Traditional DB plans were funded exclusively by employers, and provided workers with lifetime annuities based on how long they were with their employer and their final salary. DC plans, by contrast, are tax-deferred savings accounts like 401K plans which provide tax and savings incentives to both employers and employees to set aside money for retirement. The payout is determined by the amount of money contributed to the plan and the rate of return on the money invested over time. The future value of DC accounts, like savings accounts, depends both on fluctuations of the market and the worker's savvy in investing their funds wisely. A poor or misguided investment decision can decimate a worker's future retirement income. Moreover, workers with pressing and immediate financial concerns—typically women, low-income, and ethnic minority workers—may not contribute as much or frequently as is required during their working years. Consequently, just 40% of low-income workers yet more than 80% of high-income workers with DCs actually take advantage of them (Zoeckler & Silverstein, 2016). For these reasons, the historical transition from DCs to DBs as the main type of employer-provided pension has given rise to widening inequalities in pension wealth, on the basis of race, socioeconomic status, and marital status (Morrissey, 2019).

Social Security Benefits Privilege Married Persons

Social Security is a complex program, but an examination of its rules reveals how it maintains and exacerbates financial disparities on the basis of marital status. Social Security has a dual eligibility structure, meaning that it offers two paths to benefits. People can qualify for benefits either as a retired worker, or as the spouse, former spouse, or widow(er) of a retired worker (Herd, Favreault, Meyer, & Smeeding, 2018). Yet each of these paths has specific conditions that disadvantage women, persons of color, those who were married to persons with precarious employment, and those whose own employment was sporadic.

First, older adults may qualify for retired worker benefits, or Old Age, Survivors and Disability Insurance (OASDI), if they have a minimum level of earnings over 40 quarters (i.e., 40 three-month periods) or a total of 10 years of earnings. The benefits a retiree receives is based on the highest 35 years of earnings during one's working life. Second, spouse or survivor benefits are granted to those who had been married to a qualified worker for at least 10 years. When a married person reaches full retirement age, they are eligible for spousal benefits equal to one half the value of their partner's benefits. When a widow(er) reaches full retirement age, they receive benefits equal to 100% of their late spouse's benefit. However, divorced persons receive only half of their former spouse's benefit, and that benefit holds only when the marriage lasted for 10 or more years. Those who had a short-lived marriage, lasting less than 10 years, are not eligible for spouse benefits and must rely on retired worker benefits based on their earnings alone.

Older adults who qualify for both worker and spouse/survivor benefits receive just one set of benefits, whichever is higher (Iams & Tamborini, 2012). Women who have never worked for pay or who worked only sporadically, dedicating their time to childrearing rather than paid employment, might not have accrued 10 years of earnings and would have no choice but to take the spouse or survivor benefit.

Never married persons, by definition, uniformly take the worker benefit, which indirectly contributes to a considerable gap between the income levels of ever- and never-married persons. Never-married older women tended to earn considerably less than men during their working lives, a function of both discrimination and occupational sex segregation in the mid to late 20th century, where women typically were clustered in lower-paying jobs such as nurses and teachers (England, 1982). Never-married men also are disadvantaged relative to their married counterparts; current cohorts of never-married older men have lower levels of education and earnings relative to their married counterparts, due in large part to social selection. Poor physical or mental health earlier in life may have rendered them less likely to marry (Goldman, 1993; Robards, Evandrou, Falkingham, & Vlachantoni, 2012). Due in part to the well-documented earnings differential between married and never-married persons, Social Security benefits vary starkly as well. One analysis of Health and Retirement Study (HRS) data showed that the average Social Security benefit of never married men and women in 2010 was just under $12,000, whereas the mean benefit for their married counterparts slightly exceeded $22,000 (Lin et al., 2017).

Women who were in dual-earner couples may receive sparser benefits after their spouse dies, relative to those widows who had relied on the single income of a breadwinner husband. For current cohorts of older adults, women of color and low-income women are more likely than their White and higher socioeconomic status (SES) counterparts to have worked for pay throughout the childbearing years (e.g., Amott & Matthei, 1996; Fullerton, 1999). As such, they face the Social Security penalty imposed on women in dual-earner couples relative to their husband breadwinner-wife homemaker counterparts.

The math behind benefit levels is complicated, but Herd and colleagues (2018) provide a clear example to illustrate how the dual-earner couple penalty emerges. Imagine two married couples, each of whom has an annual household income of $60,000. One couple is a dual-earner family, where each spouse earns $30,000 per year. The other is a sole-breadwinner household where the husband earns $60,000 a year. When those marriages end, the wife in the sole-breadwinner household would receive a $1200 widow benefit, whereas the wife in the dual-earner household would receive just $800. As a widow, her survivor benefit would equal $800, and as a worker, her retired worker benefit would receive $800. However dual-eligibles (those eligible for benefits based on their own income as workers, or one based on their former spouse's work record) must choose just one of the two, whichever is larger. While Social Security provides a critical source of income security for nearly all older adults, the program is most beneficial for married older adults, who already enjoy a position of privilege relative to their unmarried peers.

THE IMPACT OF FAMILY STRUCTURE AND TRANSITIONS ON PHYSICAL AND EMOTIONAL WELL-BEING

Families are a critical source of comfort, companionship, and health-enhancing emotional and practical support for older adults. At the same time, family roles and responsibilities are a major source of stress in later life, with these stressors especially likely to befall older adults who have experienced social and economic disadvantages over the life course, and who lack the financial resources that may help them alter or cope with the stress-inducing situation (Pearlin, Schieman, Fazio, & Meersman, 2005). Stress is socially patterned such that less advantaged people tend to experience both a greater number of and more severe stressors. Sociologist Leonard Pearlin has described this process as stress proliferation, whereby "people exposed to a serious adversity [are] at risk for later exposure to additional adversities" while also possessing fewer material and social resources to alter the stress-inducing situation (Pearlin, Aneshensel, & Leblanc, 1997). I focus on three specific family life stressors that are especially common among those whose lives have been marked by disadvantage: bereavement, custodial grandparenthood, and caregiving.

Stress models propose that *acute events* such as the death of a spouse or child, and *chronic strains*, such as caring for a coresidential grandchild or coping with the problems that rendered one's child incapable of parenting, can threaten well-being (Pearlin et al., 2005). These experiences may be critical pathways that amplify the harmful effects of earlier adversities on health and well-being in later life. A single stressor can precede, occur alongside, or emanate from other stressors, amplifying its physical and emotional consequences. A discrete life event may give rise to chronic strains; for example, the sudden death of a spouse may trigger financial strains if that spouse had been the family's primary breadwinner (Umberson, 1992) or if the survivor is struggling to pay costly medical or funeral bills (McGarry & Schoeni, 2005). Likewise, chronic strains may precede a stressful life event; for example, an adult child's struggle with drug addiction may trigger their untimely and sudden death (Feigelman, Feigelman, & Range, 2018) and may require a bereaved older adult to serve as primary caregiver to the bereaved grandchild (Generations United, 2016). These processes of stress proliferation are especially likely to befall older adults who have experienced social and economic disadvantages over the life course, and who lack the financial resources that may help them alter or cope with the stress-inducing situation (Pearlin et al., 2005).

Family Bereavement

Socioeconomic and race disparities in mortality have widened over the past five decades, alongside rising levels of income and wealth inequality in United States (Bosworth, 2018). The gap in life expectancy between persons with higher versus lower levels of education, income, and wealth has widened since the 1980s. African Americans and persons with fewer years of education, lower levels of income, and who reside in lower-income neighborhoods consistently evidence higher rates of mortality and earlier onset of most major health conditions (including cancer, lung disease, heart disease, and diabetes) relative to Whites and their financially advantaged counterparts (Bosworth, 2018; Williams

& Sternthal, 2010). While widening mortality disparities are a critical social problem in their own right, they also mean that lower-income persons and African Americans are especially likely to experience family bereavement and its harmful consequences for health and well-being.

Family bereavement, or the death of blood, legal, or fictive kin, is considered among the most stressful of all life events, with negative consequences for one's physical and mental health (Holmes & Rahe, 1967). Familial loss, especially premature or multiple bereavements, is more common among those with limited economic resources, ethnic minorities, and women. Given women's greater life expectancy than men and their tendency to marry men slightly older than themselves, women are more likely than men to lose a spouse due to death (Federal Interagency Forum on Aging-Related Statistics, 2016).

A pathbreaking study by Umberson and colleagues (2017) concludes that elevated rates of bereavement among Blacks are an underexamined mechanism through which race and socioeconomic disparities in well-being are perpetuated. Analyzing data from the National Longitudinal Survey of Youth 1979 (NLSY79) and HRS, they find that Blacks are more likely than Whites to have survived the deaths of a mother, father, and sibling from early life through midlife. They also are more likely to have experienced child and spouse death, between midlife and old age. By age 50, Blacks are nearly twice as likely as Whites to have lost a spouse or child in the 20 years prior.

Racial disparities in mortality exist for nearly all causes, but the differential is most pronounced for violent deaths, particularly homicide. Homicide rates in the United States are among the highest of wealthy Western nations, with 4.43 violent gun deaths per 100,000 residents in the United States (compared to just .06 in the United Kingdom). Although these rates translate into small numbers in absolute terms, African Americans are especially vulnerable. Black men are 2.5 times as likely as White men to be killed by a police officer, and 1.5 times as likely to be murdered overall (Edwards, Esposito, & Lee, 2020). These violent deaths may take a profound emotional toll on the victims' aged grandparents or parents, and may deprive them of a potential source of financial support or caregiving. Homicides, in particular, are considered unjust deaths and may render older adults vulnerable to anger, an especially harmful emotional reaction as it may elevate one's risk of cardiovascular conditions (Chida & Steptoe, 2009) and "push away" those significant others who would otherwise be a source of emotional support (Keltner, Ellsworth, & Edwards, 1993).

Premature deaths, especially from stigmatized causes, also are especially likely to befall lower SES Whites relative to their higher SES counterparts. "Deaths of despair"—or deaths attributed to drug overdose (especially heroin and opioids), alcohol abuse, and suicide—increased dramatically in the late 2010s, disproportionately afflicting middle-aged high school dropouts and persons with a high school diploma only. Between 1999 and 2016, persons ages 45 to 64 of all racial and ethnic backgrounds witnessed increases in mortality rates (Woolf et al., 2018). During the same period, deaths from suicide increased by 33% (Hedegaard, Curtin, & Warner, 2020). These statistics mean that aged parents with midlife children, and retirement-age adults with slightly younger spouses or siblings, among others, are increasingly vulnerable to family bereavement due to stigmatized conditions, which may undermine the support they receive, and may intensify their feelings of guilt that they couldn't "do more" to save their loved one (Feigelman et al., 2020). Deaths related to substance use also may come at the end of a long period of family strife and financial strain, especially for costly addiction treatment programs that may deplete older adults' retirement savings (Feigelman et al., 2020). Premature deaths from homicide, suicide, and addiction exemplify the concept of stress proliferation, and are linked with prolonged symptoms of grief, depression, and symptoms similar to post-traumatic stress disorder (Kaltman & Bonanno, 2003).

Grieving a violent or untimely loss is particularly difficult, but more common losses—including the late-life loss of a spouse, parent, sibling, friend, or adult child due to chronic illness—also exact an emotional toll, although symptoms tend to return to preloss levels within 12 to 18 months post-loss (Carr & Mooney, 2021). For instance, studies generally concur that 20% to 40% of older bereaved spouses report symptoms of depression, anxiety, or grief during the first 6 months following loss before returning to preloss levels of mental health. Severe and prolonged reactions are rare, yet as many as 15% of bereaved spouses experience complicated or chronic grief; this encompasses symptoms like extreme longing for the deceased, intense emotional pain, anger, and disengagement from activities or relationships for at least 12 months following the loss (Prigerson, Vanderwerker, & Maciejewski, 2008; Shear et al., 2011). While spousal loss is linked with elevated mortality risk among widowers (Martikainen & Valkonen, 1996; Moon, Kondo, Glymour, & Subramanian, 2011), men and women do not differ dramatically with respect to most mental health symptoms (Sasson & Umberson, 2014).

Bereaved persons also tend to experience elevated symptoms of depression following the loss of an elderly parent (Scharlach & Fredriksen, 1993; Umberson, 2003), sibling (Cicirelli, 2009) or friend (d'Epinay, Cavalli, & Guillet, 2010) although these patterns do not differ dramatically on the basis of race, sex, or socioeconomic status. Child death, by contrast, is associated with more intense and long-lasting psychological symptoms among women, a function of their close ties with their children and the importance of parenting to their identities (Rogers, Floyd, Seltzer, Greenberg, & Hong, 2008). Bereavement is particularly difficult for those with the sparsest social networks and few sources of support other than the decedent. For instance, the loss of a sibling is particularly consequential for unmarried and childless older adults, who often rely on siblings to serve as their caregivers (Freedman, 1996) and their main source of social support (Steptoe, Shankar, Demakakos, & Wardle, 2013). In sum, widening economic inequalities throughout the late 20th and early 21st centuries mean that familial bereavements are especially likely to befall persons of lower SES, African Americans, and women. Moreover, the types of deaths that disadvantaged older adults are disproportionately surviving are those associated with profound symptoms of grief, including premature, violent, and stigmatized deaths, and most recently deaths from COVID-19 (Carr, Boerner, & Moorman, 2020). As such, familial bereavement is a key mechanism through which widening economic inequalities contribute to the compromised health and well-being of disadvantaged older adults.

Custodial Grandparenthood

Custodial grandparenting, or caring for grandchildren on a full-time coresidential basis, has grown increasingly common in the United States over the past five decades (Baker, Silverstein, & Putney, 2008). The share of U.S. children living in a grandparent's household has more than doubled over the past four decades, from 3% in 1970 to 7% in 2010 (Ellis & Simmons, 2012). Custodial grandparenthood is especially common among older African American women and those from economically disadvantaged backgrounds. An estimated 2.9 million older adults are currently raising their grandchildren, with African Americans and Hispanics more likely to do so, relative to Whites (Ellis & Simmons, 2012). While many custodial grandparents report that it brings them a sense of meaning, purpose, new skills, and competencies as a result of their unexpected return to the parenting role (Hayslip et al., 2019), the experience also exacts a physical, emotional, and financial toll on older adults who are already vulnerable (Choi, Sprang, & Eslinger, 2016).

The main reason that older adults are raising their grandchildren is that the middle generation, the child's parent, is not able or available to provide adequate care. Households which include a grandparent and grandchild(ren) without the middle generation are referred to as skip-generation families. The total proportion of Americans living in skip-generation households is small, although the rate is more than twice as high among Blacks (2.2%) versus other racial groups (less than 1%) (Ellis & Simmons, 2012). They also have poorer physical and economic well-being; 21% of custodial grandparents live beneath the poverty line, 25% have a disability, and 40% have provided this care for more than 5 years—rendering it a chronic strain (Ellis & Simmons, 2012).

The rising number of and racial disparities in skip-generation families and custodial grandparenting are largely a consequence of pervasive social problems that have disproportionately struck economically disadvantaged and Black families over the last four decades: the War on Drugs, mass incarceration, the HIV/AIDS epidemic, and the lingering effects of the Great Recession. Since the 1970s crackdown on illegal drugs, incarceration rates in the United States have risen dramatically, and are now among the highest in the world. Law enforcement policies like the "three strikes rule" implemented in the 1990s effectively removed large numbers of African American men and, to a lesser degree, women from their communities and into prison (Hayslip, Fruhauf, & Dolbin-MacNab, 2019).

Since the 1990s, the crack and HIV/AIDS epidemics, and extended military deployments also have disproportionately affected young men and women of color. These conditions have contributed to the premature death, incapacitation, and imprisonment of young people who might otherwise be caring for their children. In the early 2000s, many young parents—especially those with limited education and job skills—struggled to find gainful employment after losing jobs in the Great Recession (Qian, 2012). Some victims of layoffs couldn't afford their own homes or were evicted from their apartments, forcing them to place their children in a safe environment with their grandparent(s) (Turney, 2014). In the 2010s, the heroin and opioid crises have left a growing number of children (especially poorer and rural White children) either orphaned or abandoned, forcing their grandparents to step in as primary caretaker (Seelye, 2016). The psychological stress older adults experience when taking on the responsibility of custodial grandparenting is amplified by the coexisting stressors of a child's health, substance use, financial, family, or legal problems (Choi et al., 2016, Generations United, 2016).

The strains of caring for a grandchild(ren), especially against the backdrop of other family and financial stressors, may threaten older adults' well-being and are a critical mechanism contributing to health disparities. Custodial grandparents report more physical and mental health problems, poorer quality sleep, lower levels of satisfaction with the grandparenting role, poorer health behaviors, and isolation from other friends and family (Choi et al., 2016; Generations United, 2016). An analysis of HRS data found that the negative health consequences of custodial grandparenting are larger for Black grandparents, relative to their White and Hispanic counterparts (Chen et al., 2014). These harmful effects persist even when the grandparents' other risk factors, such as low income or education, are controlled (Scomeggna, 2012), although social and economic support somewhat mitigate against these effects (Chen et al., 2015).

The experience of custodial grandparenting also threatens the financial security of older adults who are already vulnerable. They must bear the costs of expenses such as clothing, furniture, extra food, school supplies, and medical bills for their grandchild(ren) (Scomeggna, 2012). Those who are of working age may experience income loss because they reduce their work hours, take a more flexible job, or quit work all together in order to manage their new role as care-taker. Reentering the labor force when their grandchild no longer requires round-the-clock care can be difficult if not impossible, given pervasive ageism in the workplace (Generations United, 2016; Meyer, 2014). These work-family strains may compound the financial and physical challenges that these vulnerable older adults faced even prior to becoming custodial caregivers.

Family Caregiving

Caregiving is a normal and expected role in later life, as older adults care for their age-peers such as a spouse, siblings, or friends, as well as the relations above (parents) or below (children or grandchildren). An estimated 40 million Americans today are providing care to a family member or friend (National Academies of Sciences, Engineering, and Medicine, 2016). However, rates of caregiving, its time intensity, perceived stressfulness, and rates of using support services vary widely on the basis of race, gender, and socioeconomic status, such that women, lower-income persons, Blacks, and Latinx persons shoulder a heavier burden than their counterparts who are male, higher-income, and White, respectively. While caregivers report benefits including a sense of meaning, purpose, the mastery of new skills, and the opportunity to "give back" to a loved one, caregivers also evidence elevated symptoms of anxiety and depression, as well as physical health decrements including an elevated risk of mortality (National Academies of Sciences, Engineering, and Medicine, 2016).

At every stage of the life course, women (even those with full-time jobs) are more likely than men to be caregivers (Sayer, 2005). These gendered patterns persist post-retirement, and converge only in very late life, at ages 85+. Women dedicate more hours per week to the care recipient, and provide care for longer time periods. According to national estimates, women spend an average of 6.1 years—nearly 10% of their adult lives—caregiving, whereas men spend just 4.1 years, or 7% of their adult life providing care to others (National Academies of Sciences, Engineering, and Medicine, 2016). Women also carry out particularly time-intensive and physically and emotionally draining tasks. Researchers classify caregiving tasks into assistance with activities of daily living (ADLs) and instrumental activities of daily living (IADLs). The former includes helping with the most basic activities that need to be accomplished each day, like dressing, toileting, and eating. The latter includes more complex activities that enable the patient to lead a full and independent life, such as cooking, driving, and managing daily medication regimes (Miller & Carfasso, 1992). Women are more likely than men to provide help with both sets of tasks, although the gender gap is a bit narrower for IADLs.

These intense time demands are a common reason why midlife and older women are more likely than men to drop out of the paid work force when they're providing care; tasks like feeding and bathing must be done every day and cannot be neglected, whereas tasks like paying bills are less frequent and urgent. Caregiving in later life, like providing childcare in young adulthood, is a key reason why women earn less during their working lives, taking a toll on their Social Security benefits, pension wealth, and risk of late-life poverty, especially after being widowed (Meyer & Herd, 2007). Labor market exits also make it more difficult to return to work, given the loss of skills during these gap times (Gonzales, Lee, & Brown, 2017).

Research on race and ethnic differences in caregiving is more limited, yet data generally show that older Blacks and Latinx invest more time in caregiving than Whites. A meta-analysis of 116 studies of racial differences in caregiving found that Blacks are more likely than Whites to help with ADLs, although no differences were detected for IADLs (Pinquart & Sorensen, 2005). Part of the reason is that Blacks, on average, suffer more numerous, frequent, and earlier onset health problems than their White counterparts. As a result, their family members and friends often are enlisted to give care at younger ages, offering assistance with basic daily tasks for long stretches of time. Older Black women are more likely than their White counterparts to provide parent care, which is particularly demanding given the parent's advanced age (Laditka and Laditka, 2001). Blacks' greater tendency to provide parent care is due in part to their lower rates of marriage, meaning that they are less likely than Whites to have a spouse available to provide time-intensive coresidential care.

Socioeconomic status differences in caregiving have garnered surprisingly little research, yet emerging evidence suggests that older adults with less education, less income, and poorer quality jobs are more likely to provide all types of care, do so for longer hours, and carry out these tasks for longer periods of time. Older adults with limited financial resources cannot pay for home health aides or the high costs of nursing home and assisted living facility supports (National Alliance of Caregivers and AARP Public Policy Institute, 2015). For older adults who are still in the workforce, juggling low-wage work and caregiving is difficult if not impossible. Workers earning an hourly wage lose pay when they take time off to provide family care. They also are unlikely to have flexible schedules, sick leave, family leave, paid vacation days, or other benefits that might help lessen the load of caregiving. For many of these older workers, the main way to manage paid work and caregiving is quitting work or reducing work hours, and spending more time on unpaid family care, which further undermines one's financial security in both the immediate and longer term (Bianchi et al., 2012).

Given these disparities in the frequency and intensity of caregiving activities, stressful caregiving may be an important mechanism that contributes to race, sex, and socioeconomic disparities in later-life well-being. Older caregivers are more likely than noncaregivers to report depression and anxiety, poorer self-rated health, sleep problems and fatigue, appetite loss, weight loss, and greater risk of cardiovascular disease, and death (Roth et al., 2013; Wolff et al., 2016). Caregiving takes an especially profound toll when one perceives their experience to be stressful; older caregivers who report high levels of psychological strain have mortality rates 50% higher than their counterparts who do not describe their caregiving as distressing (Perkins et al., 2013).

Most studies show caregiving is more harmful to physical health than emotional health, especially for older women. Caregiving duties reduce the time that one can dedicate to exercise, preparing healthy meals, sleeping 8 hours a night, complying with recommended medication schedules, and seeking care for one's own health concerns (Collins & Swartz, 2011). One study of dementia caregivers found that nearly one third neglected to take their own medications, and half did not keep their own doctors' appointments (Wang, Robinson, & Hardin, 2015). Providing physical care also can be strenuous, increasing one's risk of musculoskeletal injuries, backaches, muscle strain, scrapes, and bruises. This risk is especially dangerous for older adults who are already experiencing physical conditions like arthritis, which is more prevalent among women than men and lower SES persons relative to higher SES persons. Although Blacks and Whites have similar rates of arthritis, Blacks report higher rates of arthritis-attributed functional limitations (e.g., Barbour, Helmick, Boring, & Brady, 2017). The physical strains of intensive caregiving are amplified for those who live in subpar housing. Homes or apartments that have clutter, uneven floors and stairs, and tubs and toilets without grab bars put caregivers at risk of falls or other dangerous mishaps, especially for older caregivers with an impaired sense of balance, limited motion, and weakness due to declining muscle mass (National Academies of Sciences, Engineering, and Medicine, 2016; National Research Council, 2011). Thus, caregiving may further undermine the well-being of those older adults who already are most compromised.

CONCLUSION

I have argued that socioeconomic, race, and gender disparities in family structure have widened over the past five decades, alongside rising levels of economic
inequality. Persons whose lives are marked by greater advantage enjoy more pro-
tective family roles, further widening disparities in the economic, physical, and
emotional well-being of older adults. I described how the structure of Social Security benefits effectively privilege those who already possess the advantages of having had a long and stable marriage, exacerbating the economic disadvantages of
women and especially women of color. I then identified three family life stressors that disproportionately befall women, persons of color, and persons with
fewer socioeconomic resources—family bereavement, custodial grandparenting,
and caregiving—and further perpetuate race, gender, and socioeconomic disparities in health and well-being.

The patterns and disparities in family structures described here are projected to increase in the next three decades, as members of the large Baby Boom
and smaller Generation X cohorts reach old age. The extent to which marriage
is an institution for the privileged has intensified for recent cohorts. According
to data from the American Community Survey, 56% of upper- or middle-class
adults ages 18 to 55 are currently married, compared to just 39% of working-
class and 26% of poor people (Wilcox & Wang, 2017). Marriages also are increasingly homogamous on the basis of socioeconomic status. That means that college
graduates are marrying fellow college graduates, and high school drop-outs are
marrying other high school drop-outs, widening the gap between families who
are more or less advantaged (Schwartz, 2013). The number of Americans in dual-
earner families also is increasing. More than 60% of married couples with dependent children today are dual-earner families, compared to just 25% in 1960 (Pew,
2015). Given these demographic shifts, it is critical to the financial stability of
older adults for Social Security to alter its rules, such as reducing the 10-year marriage rule to a shorter duration, adjusting the entitlement levels for widow(er)s
and divorcees who also are retired workers, or providing an increment to never
married persons. These relatively modest adjustments will help to boost the relative financial well-being of the rising numbers of older adults whose family lives
do not conform to the mid-20th century middle-class model of marriage for life
between a homemaker and breadwinner. To date, however, policy makers have
not made efforts to restructure spouse and survivor benefits to better reflect the
contemporary realities of family life, especially for African Americans, women,
and lower-income persons.

Carefully designed policies also may mitigate against the family-related
strains that are a source of psychosocial and physical burden to vulnerable older

adults. The most straightforward policies provide practical and economic support for family caregivers, who suffer not only the physical and emotional strains of caregiving but the loss of income, wealth, and pension accumulation due to reductions in their paid employment. These practices would enhance employed older adults' capacity to give care, and would also provide supports to their family members who are a source of caregiving. The Family and Medical Leave Act (FMLA), enacted in 1993, could be expanded to better meet the needs of caregivers, especially low-income caregivers. FMLA offers up to 12 weeks of unpaid leave to workers who need to care for a family member, whether a grandchild or an ailing spouse. However, only half of all workers are covered by FMLA; those who work for smaller businesses (less than 50 employees) or have not been on the job long enough to qualify are not eligible for leave. More importantly, unpaid leave threatens the economic security of the poorest Americans and those with precarious employment; they often cannot afford to forsake their paycheck. While roughly half of U.S. workers are eligible for FMLA, rates of uptake range from just 28% among Latinx to 40% among Whites. Paid leave programs would be tremendously valuable for those forced to choose between caring for a loved one and working for pay.

Several innovative policies currently under discussion by Congress have the potential to provide some security and flexibility to caregivers. The Family and Medical Insurance Leave (FAMILY) Act would create a shared fund that makes paid leave affordable for employers of all sizes and for workers and their families. The Social Security Caregiver Credit Act would offset lost contributions during those spells when workers take their unpaid family care leave. Workers would receive a credit so that caregiving hours are included in the final calculation of their Social Security benefits. Similarly, the bipartisan proposed bill Credit for Caring Act would provide a nonrefundable federal tax credit of up to $3,000 for eligible family caregivers who work and use their own money to help care for a loved one. Although the future of this proposed legislation is uncertain, policy makers from both sides of the aisle agree that some forms of public support for caregivers is critical (Carr, 2019). Older adults will account for an unprecedented 21% of the U.S. population by the year 2030, with their ranks projected to top 74 million. The needs of these older adults and the family members that care for or are cared for by then must be addressed, and strategic federal policies are a critical first step toward ensuring that all older adults—including those who have faced cumulative disadvantages—have the opportunity to live with dignity and comfort.

REFERENCES

Amott, T., & Matthaei, J. (1996). *Race, gender, and work: A multicultural economic history of women in the U.S.* Boston, MA: South End Press.

Angel, J. L., Montez, J. K., & Angel, R. J. (2011). A window of vulnerability: Health insurance coverage among women 55 to 64 years of age. *Women's Health Issues, 21*(1), 6–11.

Baker, L. A., Silverstein, M., & Putney, N. M. (2008). Grandparents raising grandchildren in the United States: Changing family forms, stagnant social policies. *Journal of Societal & Social Policy, 7*, 53–69.

Barbour, K. E., Helmick, C. G., Boring, M. A., & Brady, T. J. (2017). Vital signs: Prevalence of doctor-diagnosed arthritis and arthritis-attributable activity limitation—United States, 2013–2015. *Morbidity and Mortality Weekly Reports, 66*, 246–253.

Bianchi, S. M. (1999). Feminization and juvenilization of poverty: Trends, relative risks, causes, and consequences. *Annual Review of Sociology, 25*(1), 307–333.

Bianchi, S. M., Sayer, L. C., Milkie, M. A., & Robinson, J. P. (2012). Housework: Who did, does or will do it, and how much does it matter? *Social Forces, 91*(1), 55–63.

Bosworth, B. (2018). Increasing disparities in mortality by socioeconomic status. *Annual Review of Public Health, 39*, 237–251.

Brown, S. L., Lin, I. F., Hammersmith, A. M., & Wright, M. R. (2016). Later life marital dissolution and repartnership status: A national portrait. *The Journals of Gerontology: Series B, 73*(6), 1032–1042.

Carr, D. (2019). *Golden years? Social inequality in later life.* New York, NY: Russell Sage Foundation.

Carr, D., Boerner, K., & Moorman, S. (2020). Bereavement in the time of Coronavirus: Unprecedented challenges demand novel interventions. *Journal of Aging & Social Policy*, 1–7. doi:10.1080/08959420.2020.1764320

Carr, D., & Mooney, H. (2021). Bereavement in later life. Chapter 15 in K. Ferraro & D. Carr (Eds.), *Handbook of aging and the social sciences* (9th ed.). New York, NY: Academic Press.

Carr, D., & Springer, K. W. (2010). Advances in families and health research in the 21st century. *Journal of Marriage and Family, 72*(3), 743–761.

Carr, D., & Utz, R. L. (2020). Families in later life: A decade in review. *Journal of Marriage and Family, 82*(1), 346–363.

Chen, F., Mair, C. A., Bao, L., & Yang, Y. C. (2015). Race/ethnic differentials in the health consequences of caring for grandchildren for grandparents. *Journals of Gerontology Series B: Psychological Sciences and Social Sciences, 70*(5), 793–803.

Cherlin, A. J. (2010). *The marriage-go-round: The state of marriage and the family in America today.* New York, NY: Vintage.

Chida, Y., & Steptoe, A. (2009). The association of anger and hostility with future coronary heart disease: A meta-analytic review of prospective evidence. *Journal of the American College of Cardiology, 53*(11), 936–946.

Choi, M., Sprang, G., & Eslinger, J. G. (2016). Grandparents raising grandchildren. *Family & Community Health, 39*(2), 120–128.

Cicirelli, V. G. (2009). Sibling death and death fear in relation to depressive symptomatology in older adults. *Journals of Gerontology Series B: Psychological and Social Sciences*, 64(1), 24–32.

Cohen, P. N., & Pepin, J. R. (2018). Unequal marriage markets: Sex ratios and first marriage among Black and White women. *Socius, 4.* https://doi.org/10.1177/2378023118791084

Collins, L. G., & Swartz, K. (2011). Caregiver care. *American Family Physician*, 83(11), 1309–1307.

Congressional Budget Office. (2019). The *distribution of household income, 2016.* Washington, DC: Author. Retrieved from https://www.cbo.gov/system/files/2019-07/55413-CBO-distribution-of-household-income-2016.pdf

Hedegaard, H., Curtin, S. C., & Warner, M. (2020). Increase in suicide mortality in the United States, 1999–2018. NCHS Data Brief, No. 362, DHHS Publication, No. 2020–1209. Washington, DC: NCHS.

d'Epinay, C. J. L., Cavalli, S., & Guillet, L. A. (2010). Bereavement in very old age: Impact on health and relationships of the loss of a spouse, a child, a sibling, or a close friend. *OMEGA Journal of Death and Dying*, 60(4), 301–325.

Dewilde, C. (2008). Divorce and the housing movements of owner-occupiers: A European comparison. *Housing Studies*, 23(6), 809–832.

Edwards, F., Esposito, M. H., & Lee, H. (2018). Risk of police-involved death by race/ethnicity and place, United States, 2012–2018. *American Journal of Public Health*, 108(9), 1241–1248.

Ellis, R. R., & Simmons, T. (2012). *Coresident grandparents and their grandchildren. Current Population Reports* (P20-576). Washington, DC: U.S. Census Bureau.

England, P. (1982). The failure of human capital theory to explain occupational sex segregation. *Journal of Human Resources*, 17, 358–370.

England, P., & McClintock, E. A. (2009). The gendered double standard of aging in US marriage markets. *Population and Development Review*, 35(4), 797–816.

Fan, J. X., & Zick, C. D. (2006). Expenditure flows near widowhood. *Journal of Family and Economic Issues*, 27(2), 335–353.

Federal Interagency Forum on Aging-Related Statistics. (2016). *Older Americans 2016: Key indicators of well-being.* Washington, DC: U.S. Government Printing Office.

Feigelman, W., Feigelman, B., & Range, L. M. (2020). Grief and healing trajectories of drug–death–bereaved parents. *OMEGA—Journal of Death and Dying*, 80(4), 629–647. doi:10.1177/0030222818754669

Freedman, V. (1996). Family structure and the risk of nursing home admission. *Journals of Gerontology Series B: Psychological and Social Sciences*, 51(2), S61–69.

Fullerton, H. N., Jr. (1999). Labor force participation: 75 years of change, 1950–98 and 1998–2025. *Monthly Labor Review*, 122, 3–12.

Generations United. (2016). *State of grandfamilies 2016. Raising the children of the opioid epidemic: Solutions and support for grandfamilies.* Washington, DC: Author. Retrieved fromhttps://dl2.pushbulletusercontent.com/qdCNUO2JMMZKzKRjyIlwbgjMtf39xkKa/16-Report-SOGF-Final.pdf

Gibson-Davis, C. M., & Percheski, C. (2018). Children and the elderly: Wealth inequality among America's dependents. *Demography, 55,* 1009–1032.

Goldman, N. (1993). Marriage selection and mortality patterns: Inferences and fallacies. *Demography, 30,* 189–208.

Gonzales, E., Lee, Y., & Brown, C. (2017). Back to work? Not everyone. Examining the longitudinal relationships between informal caregiving and paid work after formal retirement. *The Journals of Gerontology: Series B, 72*(3), 532–539.

Harris, T. F., & Yelowitz, A. (2018). Racial disparities in life insurance coverage. *Applied Economics, 50*(1), 94–107.

Hayslip, B., Jr., Fruhauf, C. A., & Dolbin-MacNab, M. L. (2019). Grandparents raising grandchildren: What have we learned over the past decade? *The Gerontologist, 59*(3), e152–e163.

Hayslip, B., Jr., Glover, R. J., Harris, B. E., Miltenberger, P. B., Baird, A., & Kaminski, P. L. (2009). Perceptions of custodial grandparents among young adults. *Journal of Intergenerational Relationships, 7*(2–3), 209–224.

Herd, P., Favreault, M., Meyer, M. H., & Smeeding, T. M. (2018). A targeted minimum benefit plan: A new proposal to reduce poverty among older social security recipients. *RSF: The Russell Sage Foundation Journal of the Social Sciences, 4*(2), 74–90.

Holmes, T. H., & Rahe, R. H. (1967). The social readjustment rating scale. *Journal of Psychosomatic Research, 11,* 213–218.

Iams, H. M., & Tamborini, C. R. (2012). The implications of marital history change on women's eligibility for social security wife and widow benefits, 1990–2009. *Social Security Bulletin, 72,* 23–38.

Kaltman, S., & Bonanno, G. A. (2003). Trauma and bereavement: Examining the impact of sudden and violent deaths. *Journal of Anxiety Disorders, 17*(2), 131–147.

Keltner, D., Ellsworth, P. C., & Edwards, K. (1993). Beyond simple pessimism: Effects of sadness and anger on social perception. *Journal of Personality and Social Psychology, 64,* 740–752.

Laditka, J. N., & Laditka, S. B. (2001). Adult children helping older parents: Variations in likelihood and hours by gender, race, and family role. *Research on Aging, 23*(4), 429–456.

Leopold, T. (2018). Gender differences in the consequences of divorce: A study of multiple outcomes. *Demography, 55*(3), 769–797.

Lin, I. F., Brown, S. L., & Hammersmith, A. M. (2017). Marital biography, social security receipt, and poverty. *Research on Aging, 39*(1), 86–110.

Livingston, G., Parker, K., & Ruhal, M. (2014). *The demographics of remarriage. Four-in-ten couples are saying "I Do," again.* Washington, DC: Pew. Retrieved from https://www.pewresearch.org/wp-content/uploads/sites/3/2014/11/2014-11-14_remarriage-final.pdf

Lundberg, S., Pollak, R. A., & Stearns, J. (2016). Family inequality: Diverging patterns in marriage, cohabitation, and childbearing. *The Journal of Economic Perspectives, 30*(2), 79–101.

Manduca, R. (2018). Income inequality and the persistence of racial economic disparities. *Sociological Science*, 5, 182–205.

Martikainen, P., & Valkonen, T. (1996). Mortality after the death of a spouse: Rates and causes of death in a large Finnish cohort. *American Journal of Public Health*, 86(8), 1087–1093.

McGarry, K., & Schoeni, R. F. (2005). Widow(er) poverty and out-of-pocket medical expenditures near the end of life. *The Journals of Gerontology Series B: Psychological Sciences and Social Sciences*, 60(3), S160–S168.

Meyer, M. H. (2014). *Grandmothers at work: Juggling families and jobs*. New York, NY: New York University Press.

Meyer, M. H., & Herd, P. (2007). *Market friendly or family friendly? The state and gender inequality in old age*. New York, NY: Russell Sage Foundation.

Miller, B., & Cafasso, L. (1992). Gender differences in caregiving: Fact or artifact? *The Gerontologist*, 32(4), 498–507.

Moon, J. R., Kondo, N., Glymour, M. M., & Subramanian, S. V. (2011). Widowhood and mortality: A meta-analysis. *PloS One*, 6(8), e23465.

Morrissey, M. (2019, December). *The state of American retirement savings*. Washington, DC: Economic Policy Institute. Retrieved from https://www.epi.org/publication/the-state-of-american-retirement-savings/

National Academies of Sciences, Engineering, and Medicine. (2016). *Families caring for an aging America*. Washington, DC: The National Academies Press.

National Alliance of Caregivers and AARP Public Policy Institute. (2015). *Caregiving in the U.S.* Washington, DC: Author.

National Research Council. (2011). *Health care comes home: The human factors*. Washington, DC: National Academies Press.

Painter, J. A., Elliott, S. J., & Hudson, S. (2009). Falls in community-dwelling adults aged 50 years and older prevalence and contributing factors. *Journal of Allied Health*, 38(4), 201–207.

Pearlin, L. I., Aneshensel, C. S., & LeBlanc, A. J. (1997). The forms and mechanisms of stress proliferation: The case of AIDS caregivers. *Journal of Health and Social Behavior*, 38(3), 223.

Pearlin, L. I., Schieman, S., Fazio, E. M., & Meersman, S. C. (2005). Stress, health, and the life course: Some conceptual perspectives. *Journal of Health and Social Behavior*, 46(2), 205–219.

Perkins, M., Howard, V. J., Wadley, V. G., Crowe, M., Safford, M. M., Haley, W. E., ... Roth, D. L. (2013). Caregiving strain and all-cause mortality: Evidence from the REGARDS study. *Journals of Gerontology Series B: Psychological Sciences and Social Sciences*, 68(4), 504–512.

Pew Research Center. (2015, December 17). *Parenting in America*. Washington, DC: Author.

Pickett, K. E., & Wilkinson, R. G. (2015). Income inequality and health: A causal review. *Social Science & Medicine*, 128, 316–326.

Piketty, T. (2014). *Capital in the 21st century*. Cambridge, MA: Harvard University Press.

Pinquart, M., & Sörensen, S. (2005). Ethnic differences in stressors, resources, and psychological outcomes of family caregiving: A meta-analysis. *The Gerontologist, 45*(1), 90–106.

Prigerson, H. G., Vanderwerker, L. C., & Maciejewski, P. K. (2008). A case for inclusion of prolonged grief disorder in DSM-V. In M. Stroebe, R. O. Hansson, H. Schut, & W. Stroebe (Eds.), *Handbook of bereavement research and practice: 21st century perspectives* (pp. 165–186). Washington, DC: American Psychological Association (APA) Press.

Qian, Z. (2012). *During the Great Recession, more young adults lived with parents.* Census Brief prepared for Project US2010, Washington, DC. Retrieved from http://www.russellsage.org/sites/all/files/US2010/US2010_Qian_20120801.pdf

Raley, R. K., Sweeney, M. M., & Wondra, D. (2015). The growing racial and ethnic divide in US marriage patterns. *The Future of Children/Center for the Future of Children, the David and Lucile Packard Foundation. 25*(2), 89.

Rhee, N. (2013). *Race and retirement insecurity in the United States.* Washington, DC: National Institute on Retirement Security.

Robards, J., Evandrou, M., Falkingham, J., & Vlachantoni, A. (2012). Marital status, health and mortality. *Maturitas, 73*(4), 295–299.

Rogers, C. H., Floyd, F. J., Seltzer, M. M., Greenberg, J., & Hong, J. (2008). Long-term effects of the death of a child on parents' adjustment in midlife. *Journal of Family Psychology, 22*(2), 203–211.

Romig, K., & Sherman, A. (2016). *Social Security keeps 22 million Americans out of poverty: A state-by-state analysis.* Washington, DC: Center on Budget and Policy Priorities.

Roth, D. L., Haley, W. E., Hovater, M., Perkins, M., Wadley, V. G., & Judd, S. (2013). Family caregiving and all-cause mortality: Findings from a population-based propensity-matched analysis. *American Journal of Epidemiology, 178*(10), 1571–1578.

Sasson, I., & Umberson, D. J. (2014). Widowhood and depression: New light on gender differences, selection, and psychological adjustment. *Journals of Gerontology Series B: Psychological and Social Sciences, 69*(1), 135–145.

Sawhill, I., & Venator, J. (2015). *Is there a shortage of marriageable men? Center on children and families.* Washington, DC: Brookings. Retrieved from https://pdfs.semanticscholar.org/a051/eb28b75a12253034006a1b7120dbb22e0cb0.pdf

Sayer, L. C. (2005). Gender, time and inequality: Trends in women's and men's paid work, unpaid work and free time. *Social Forces, 84*(1), 285–303.

Scharlach, A. E., & Fredriksen, K. I. (1993). Reactions to the death of a parent during midlife. *OMEGA, 27*, 307–319.

Schwartz, C. R. (2013). Trends and variation in assortative mating: Causes and consequences. *Annual Review of Sociology, 39*, 451–470.

Scommegna, P. (2012, March). *More US children raised by grandparents.* Washington, DC: Population Reference Bureau.

Seelye, K. Q. (2016, May). Children of heroin crisis find refuge in grandparents' arms. *The New York Times.* Retrieved from http://www.nytimes.com/interactive/2016/05/05/us/grandparents-heroin-impact-kids.html

Semyonov, M., Lewin-Epstein, N., & Bridges, W. P. (2011). Explaining racial disparities in access to employment benefits. *Ethnic and Racial Studies, 34*(12), 2069–2095.

Shafer, K., & James, S. L. (2013). Gender and socioeconomic status differences in first and second marriage formation. *Journal of Marriage and Family, 75*(3), 544–564.

Shear, M. K., Simon, N., Wall, M., Zisook, S., Neimeyer, R., Duan, N., . . . Keshaviah, A. (2011). Complicated grief and related bereavement issues for DSM-5. *Depression and Anxiety, 28*(2), 103–117.

Smith, K. J., & Victor, C. (2019). Typologies of loneliness, living alone and social isolation, and their associations with physical and mental health. *Ageing & Society, 39*(8), 1709–1730.

Smock, P. J., Manning, W. D., & Gupta, S. (1999). The effect of marriage and divorce on women's economic well-being. *American Sociological Review, 64*, 794–812.

Smock, P. J., & Schwartz, C. R. (2020). The demography of families: A review of patterns and change. *Journal of Marriage and Family, 82*(1), 9–34.

Steptoe, A., Shankar, A., Demakakos, P., & Wardle, J. (2013). Social isolation, loneliness, and all-cause mortality in older men and women. *Proceedings of the National Academy of Sciences, 110*(15), 5797–5801.

Stoltzfus, E. R. (2016). Defined contribution retirement plans: Who has them and what do they cost? *Beyond the Numbers, 5*(17). Washington, DC: Bureau of Labor Statistics.

Tach, L. M., & Eads, A. (2015). Trends in the economic consequences of marital and cohabitation dissolution in the United States. *Demography, 52*(2), 401–432.

Turney, K. (2014). Incarceration and social inequality: Challenges and directions for future research. *The Annals of the American Academy of Political and Social Science, 651*(1), 97–101.

Umberson, D. (1992). Gender, marital status and the social control of health behavior. *Social Science & Medicine, 34*(8), 907–917.

Umberson, D. (2003). *Death of a parent: Transition to a new adult identity.* New York, NY: Cambridge University Press.

Umberson, D., Olson, J. S., Crosnoe, R., Liu, H., Pudrovska, T., & Donnelly, R. (2017). Death of family members as an overlooked source of racial disadvantage in the United States. *Proceedings of the National Academy of Sciences, 114*(5), 915–920.

U.S. Bureau of the Census. (2015). *Current population survey, 2015 annual social and economic supplement.* Washington, DC: U.S. Government Printing Office. Retrieved from ftp://ftp2.census.gov/programs-surveys/cps/techdocs/cpsmar15.pdf

Wang, X., Robinson, K. M., & Hardin, H. K. (2015). The impact of caregiving on caregivers' medication adherence and appointment keeping. *Western Journal of Nursing Research, 37*(12), 1548–1562.

Wilcox, W. B., & Wang, W. (2017). *The marriage divide: How and why working class-families are more fragile today.* Washington, DC: AEI/Brookings Institute. Retrieved from http://www.aei.org/wp-content/uploads/2017/09/The-Marriage-Divide.pdf

Williams, D. R., & Sternthal, M. (2010). Understanding racial-ethnic disparities in health: Sociological contributions. *Journal of Health and Social Behavior, 51*, S15–S27.

Wilson, W. J. (1987). *The truly disadvantaged: The inner city, the underclass, and public policy.* Chicago, IL: University of Chicago.

Wolff, J. L., Spillman, B. C., Freedman, V. A., & Kasper, J. D. (2016). A national profile of family and unpaid caregivers who assist older adults with health care activities. *JAMA Internal Medicine, 176*(3), 372–379.

Woolf, S. H., Chapman, D. A., Buchanich, J. M., Bobby, K. J., Zimmerman, E. B., & Blackburn, S. M. (2018). Changes in midlife death rates across racial and ethnic groups in the United States: Systematic analysis of vital statistics. *BMJ, 362*, k3096.

Wu, Z., & Schimmele, C. M. (2005). Repartnering after first union disruption. *Journal of Marriage and Family, 67*(1), 27–36.

Zoeckler, J. M., & Silverstein, M. (2016). Work and retirement. In M. H. Meyer & E. A. Daniele (Eds.), *Gerontology: Changes, challenges, and solutions: Changes, challenges, and solutions* (pp. pp. 161–190). Santa Barbara, CA: Praeger Publishers.

CHAPTER 4

Increasing Risks, Costs, and Retirement Income Inequality

Christian E. Weller and Katherine Newman

ABSTRACT

Over the past three decades, retirement inequality has grown more serious for both low-income and middle-income families. Both slow wage growth and modest (to no) upward economic mobility have made it hard for people to save for their retirement. At the same time, economic risks have become more widespread and many costs have risen, making it harder for families to save. Key risks include earnings instability, the growth of defined contribution retirement savings accounts, home equity as a retirement savings vehicle, and unpaid family caregiving. Each of these risks creates its own obstacles for families to save for their future. Families also face rising costs, especially for healthcare and education that put additional pressures on their budgets and make it harder for them to put money away for the future. We summarize the evidence on the link between key risks and costs, on the one hand, and household savings, on the other. They remain understudied contributors to retirement income inequality, however. We thus point to a number of open research questions. Answering these questions could provide better insights on the distribution of the relevant risks. These answers will give policymakers a sense of the target audiences if they want to create more economic stability prior to retirement. They could also offer more evidence on the causal mechanisms by which more income volatility lowers retirement savings. This could further help identify pathways for new policy interventions to help people save more for their retirement.

© 2020 Springer Publishing Company
http://dx.doi.org/10.1891/0198-8794.40.69

INTRODUCTION

Retirement security has always been unequally distributed. When the risks become excessive and millions of retirees face economic hardship, policy makers respond with social insurance protections such as Social Security and Medicare that mitigate some of the worst risks. These solutions are no longer sufficient.

Over the past three decades, retirement inequality has grown more serious and the risks involved are spreading to a larger number of American families. It is virtually assured that they will have to make substantial and painful spending cuts, be unable to see a doctor or pay the rent, and face the prospect that they will live out their days in poverty and material hardship. But inequality—a force we have long recognized at play among prime age workers—will translate into hardship and indignity for some and the total absence of financial concerns for others.

Retirement insecurity is no longer a problem for the poor alone. Many middle-income families will also face economic uncertainty at older ages. This trend is likely to continue since inequality in retirement wealth is greater for younger families today than it was for previous generations at similar stages in their lives.

Many forces related to economic inequality have conspired to make it so. Slow wage growth and modest (to no) upward economic mobility have made it hard for people to save for their retirement. At the same time, economic risks have become more widespread and many costs have risen, making it harder for families to save, while adding costs for retirees. Wages have become less stable not just for low-wage workers but also for many middle-income employees. The earnings patterns of Millennials faltered as the toll of the Great Recession dismantled career pathways and put pressure on their parents to step in and help, thus diminishing the capacity for Baby Boomers and Gen Xers to save for retirement. Most low-wage workers have no work-related retirement benefits. Middle-income workers who do face more financial risks with their retirement savings now than in the past.

Low-income and middle-income families have relied on home equity as a form of insurance for the future, which exposes them to additional financial risks when housing markets falter. This became abundantly clear during the Great Recession from 2007 to 2009.

Families across the income spectrum are responsible for the support of children well into their own adulthood, posing additional obstacles to saving for retirement. Similarly, the need to support elders puts a growing squeeze on Boomer savings. Moreover, costs for key items, especially healthcare and education typically outpace wages as well as retirement incomes, making it simultaneously harder and more necessary to save.

Because income volatility and accelerating costs increases put pressure on household budgets, families have been raiding their savings to cover their bills when income fluctuates due to layoffs, reduced hours, and unanticipated caregiving demands. At the same time, families have to spend more to pay for their own healthcare and their children's education. This pincer movement translates into either more debt or diminished savings. These burdens can become so complex that families avoid planning for the future altogether. The stress involved can be overwhelming.

In this review, we summarize the evidence on the link between key risks and costs, on the one hand, and household savings, on the other. We consider how increasing volatility and higher costs have contributed to the income inequality among seniors. Each of these factors impedes retirement savings for many lower-income and middle-income families. We conclude each section with a set of unanswered research questions which, we argue, should form a research agenda if we are to fully understand the dynamics of inequality in retirement.

How Do Less Stable Working Lives Translate Into Fewer Retirement Savings?

Analyses of retirement wealth and its distribution that we discuss in the following do not systematically incorporate economic risks that can disrupt retirement savings during prime working years. Income volatility has grown over time and thus contributed to more retirement inequality. Low income growth and lack of mobility already translates into old-age economic insecurity (Government Accountability Office, 2019). Greater income volatility during people's careers further exacerbates this uncertainty.

Income inequality has grown over much of the past 40 years. Piketty et al. (2017) conclude that the average income for the bottom half of the income distribution was flat between 1980 and 2014; even worse, he records a decline of 25% for those in the bottom 20% of the income distribution. In comparison, incomes have grown by 40% for adults between the median and the 90th percentile and risen very sharply at 120% for those in the top 10% of the income distribution (Piketty et al., 2017).

At the same time, **income mobility** has fallen (Chetty, 2016; Chetty et al., 2014, 2017; Katz & Krueger, 2017). For example, Raj Chetty and his co-authors (2016) find that 90% of children born in 1940 eventually earned more than their parents did, but only 50% of children born in 1980 did. As a result, economic mobility appears to be less in the United States than in other developed countries such as the United Kingdom, Denmark, and Canada (Chetty, 2016). Katz and Krueger (2017) confirm these findings in their review. The income distribution has become "sticky," leading families to persist in their positions at the top and the bottom, a phenomenon that has translated into greater wealth inequality and thus increasing retirement income inequality.

Increasing **income volatility** is a third contributing factor to retirement wealth inequality. Dynan, Elmendorf, and Sichel (2012) find that income volatility has grown from the 1970s to late 2000s. After 2000, lower-income households had a 12% chance of income drops that were greater than 50% of their income, compared to 7% in the 1970s (Dynan et al., 2012). Hardy and Ziliak (2014) similarly find increasing income volatility at the bottom, but also at the top of the income distribution. Underlying changes in income volatility appear to be increases in earnings volatility for men (Dahl et al., 2007; Gottschalk, Moffitt, Katz, & Dickens, 1994; Haider, 2001; Shin and Solon, 2011; Ziliak et al., 2011) and women (Ziliak et al., 2011).

Instability in earnings has many sources, but among them are irregular work schedules, unemployment spells and contingent pay such as tips, bonuses and commissions (Board of Governors, Federal Reserve System, 2014). Industries like retail and restaurants, which have grown over time (Golden, 2015; Morduch & Schneider, 2017), are particularly prone to this erratic pattern.

Families experiencing more income volatility find it more difficult to build wealth for retirement for a number of reasons. They have to prepare for shocks by putting less money towards risky (but potentially more valuable) assets, most notably stocks (Gollier & Pratt, 1996; Kimball, 1993; Pratt & Zeckhauser, 1987). They increase precautionary savings (Cagetti, 2003; Carroll & Samwick, 1998; Gourinchas & Parker, 2001; Guiso et al., 1992; Guiso et al., 1996; Hochguertel, 2003). A widening gap between those who do and do not experience income volatility contributes to growing wealth inequality as those affected hold more cash and other liquid assets that earn lower rates of return.

Increased income volatility leads families to inadvertently follow a "buy high, sell low" strategy for their investments. Earnings fall when the economy weakens and stock prices drop. Lower stock prices present buying opportunities, but workers cannot take advantage of them because they have lower incomes. Many workers may actually need to sell some of their stocks when prices are low to gain access to income during a downturn. When the economy improves again, it takes time for earnings to go back up, while stock prices rise more quickly, leading workers to buy stocks at higher prices. Pro-cyclical income volatility thus reduces returns on families' investments and contributes to retirement income inequality by gender, race, and education (Seligman & Wenger, 2006; Weller & Wenger, 2009).

Families with more unstable incomes also become more risk averse. They are less willing to invest their money for the longer term (Benito, 2006; Gonyea, 2007; Orel et al., 2004; Weller, 2018). The result is again fewer investment in potentially riskier investments that also offer the chance of higher returns and also fewer savings in general, both of which contribute to more wealth inequality.

Further, income volatility can cause acute stress (Rohde et al., 2016; Sinclair & Cheung, 2016) that contributes to lower savings (Porcelli & Delgado, 2009). People under pressure rely more on automated decision-making processes and thus miss saving and investment opportunities that require active decision-making (Porcelli & Delgado, 2009). They may be less likely to sign up for a retirement savings account at work and miss out on employer savings matches, for instance. Growing income volatility sets up more hurdles to saving for retirement, contributing to wealth inequality.

The existing research on the link between income volatility and wealth inequality leaves some questions unaddressed. The psychological dimension of financial risks and insecurity, particularly the acute stress that results, are often not incorporated in economic models of saving behavior. Stress, though, can worsen other well-known barriers to saving. Moreover, it is likely that income volatility has different savings effects by gender, race, and ethnicity because of other correlated risks. A better understanding of the exact links between volatility and wealth inequality could help refine policy interventions to help families save more.

Is There Really a Retirement Crisis?

As income inequality has risen, income mobility has declined and income volatility has grown. Accordingly, retirement preparedness has gone down. The exact proportion of working families who will face retirement insecurity differs between data sets and measurement methods, but there is no doubt that a sizeable minority of working families have not saved enough to avoid deep and painful spending cuts.

This share has grown over time and is likely to worsen in succeeding generations. Moreover, the likelihood of retirement insecurity is greater for women than men, among people with less education, and among people of color. Researchers use two separate approaches to assess whether working families will be ready for a secure retirement. Both approaches relate people's total sources of future retirement income—Social Security benefits, defined benefit pensions, and all savings—to their incomes prior to retirement.

One method considers whether families will be able to maintain similar spending levels in retirement as they did during their working lives (Ameriks & Utkus, 2006; Bernheim, 1997; Biggs & Springstead, 2008; Boskin & Shoven, 1984; Ellis, Munnell, & Eschtruth, 2014; Engen, Engen, & Engen, 2005; Engen, Gale, Uccello, Carroll, & Laibson 2005; Gale, Scholz, & Seshadri, 2009;

Gustman & Steinmeier, 1999; Haveman, Holden, Romanov, & Wolfe, 2005; Lusardi & Mitchell, 2011; Moore & Mitchell, 2000; Munnell et al., 2006; Palmer, 2002; Rhee, 2013; Rhee & Boive, 2015; Scholz, Seshadri, & Khitatrakun, 2006; VanDerhei, 2015; Warshawsky & Ameriks, 2000). This approach defines retirement income adequacy as a minimum ratio of retirement income relative to pre-retirement earnings. A family is deemed adequately prepared if their expected retirement income is greater than a minimum share—typically 70% to 85%—of a family's income before retirement.[1]

We can approximate this approach by looking at household wealth-to-income ratios for nonretirees. Rising median wealth-to-income ratios would suggest improving retirement adequacy and potentially declining inequality, while the opposite would be true for declining ratios.[2] Even stagnant wealth-to-income ratios would suggest increasing retirement income shortfalls since successive generations face greater costs.

Figure 4.1 shows the median wealth-to-income ratios for seven different age groups among nonretirees from 1989 to 2016. Wealth is the difference between all assets, including the imputed wealth of defined benefit (DB) pensions, minus all debt (Sabelhaus & Henriques, 2019). The median wealth-to-income ratio for families from 55 to 64 years declined from 2001 to 2010 before making a small recovery (Figure 4.1). The age group closest to retirement is thus worse prepared now than it was two decades ago.

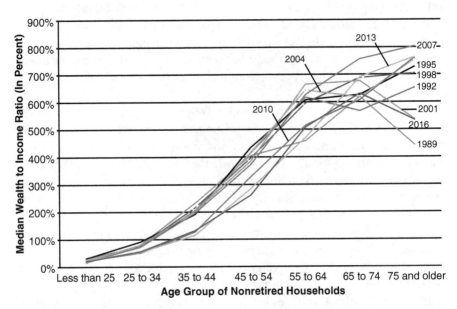

FIGURE 4.1 Median wealth-to-income ratios for nonretired households by age and year, 1989 to 2016.

An alternative approach to retirement income adequacy measures whether retirees will have enough income to avoid poverty (Butrica et al., 2010; Ameriks & Utkus, 2006; Haveman et al., 2005; Love et al., 2009) and material hardships (Center for Social and Demographic Research on Aging, 2017; Mutchler et al., 2016, 2017a, 2017b; Weller & Wolff, 2005; Wolff, 2015).

These two approaches complement each other in informing public policy. The replacement rate shows which population groups will likely have to cut spending in retirement. Policy makers could thus target policy interventions to boost savings and income replacement programs for those families and retirees. DB pensions and defined contribution (DC) savings accounts such as 401(k) plans tie savings to earnings and are anchored in this approach. In comparison, comparing retirement income to poverty and material hardships shows which groups of retirees won't be able to pay for basic necessities. This informs the design of social programs to cover basic costs such as food, housing, and healthcare in old age. Social Security's retirement benefits reflect both approaches as they offer relatively more generous benefits to workers with lower lifetime earnings than for higher lifetime earners.

Both methods lead to the same dismal conclusion: inequality by age, race, ethnicity, and gender is pronounced among retirees.

How Well Are Americans Prepared for Retirement?

Boston College's Center for Retirement Research (CRR) has developed a useful indicator of how well working families are prepared for retirement: the National Retirement Risk Index (NRRI). For 2016, its estimate shows that 50% of working families are at risk of being unable to maintain their spending in retirement (Munnell et al., 2018). Similarly, Wolff (2015) projects that 51% of households near retirement—47 to 64 years old—in 2010 will be unable to replace 75% of their preretirement income in retirement, somewhat lower than the 53% of all working families estimated for that year by Munnell et al. (2018).

Other estimates put the share of working families that are ill prepared much higher. Rhee and Boivie (2015) estimate that 66.2% of working families did not meet financial industry standards for a secure retirement, using the same data source as the CRR's NRRI does, which shows only a shortfall of 53% of working families for that year (Munnell et al., 2018).

On the other hand, some studies see a less dire situation. William Gale and his co-authors (2009), for example, concluded that 26% of households did not have enough savings in 2004 to maintain their spending in retirement. They use a different data set and, more importantly, different assumptions about retiree spending behavior than Munnell et al. (2018) who estimated a share of 45% of working age families at risk of an insecure retirement for 2004 (Munnell et al.,

2018). Butrica, Smith, and Iams (2012) use a simulation model to show that conditional on age, between 35% and 43% of those reaching retirement at 67 will be able to replace less than 75% of their preretirement earnings in 2012, below the 53% estimated by Munnell et al. (2018).

The second approach to measuring retirement security also shows widespread economic insecurity among older households. The Elder Economic Security Standard™, for instance, shows that 53% of households 65 years old and older did not have incomes high enough to pay for basic things like health-care and housing in 2016 (Mutchler et al., 2016). Weller and Wolff (2005) find that 29.7% of households between the ages of 47 and 64 years old had expected retirement incomes of less than twice the poverty line based on their wealth in 2001.

Regardless of which studies we examined, the problem of income insufficiency is real and growing and will impact the standard of living of retirees, though those with lower earnings during their prime years (which includes women and minorities) will feel the bite more deeply.

Do Retirees Spend Less Money Than Workers?

Retirement insecurity expresses itself in limitations on spending.[3] The seriousness of the problem differs depending on assumptions about spending behavior.[4]

If retirees spend less, they will need less in the way of savings. Researchers who forecast more modest shortfalls, including Gale et al. (2009), assume that retirees will cut back their spending because their household size is smaller since children have left home, the average family size has been declining, and deceased spouses no longer require support. Several researchers indeed find a sharp drop in spending when people retire (Banks, Blundell, & Tanner, 1998, Bernheim, Skinner, & Weinberg, 2001, Haider & Stephens, 2007; Hurd & Rohwedder, 2003; Schwerdt, 2005). Others, though, argue that retirees only cut some spending (such as restaurant meals) because they have more free time to prepare meals (Aguiar & Hurst, 2005, 2013; Hurst, 2007). Retirees do not spend less on non-food consumption (Aguila, Attanasio, & Meghir, 2011).

These studies only consider spending changes at the point of retirement rather than over the years that follow. Taking the longer view changes the picture. David Blanchett (2013) shows that retiree spending declines at first, but then increases again, potentially because of rapidly rising healthcare costs, a risk that is commonly ignored when looking only at the transition into retirement. Still, a large number of people die with substantial savings leftover, suggesting that they spent less in retirement, perhaps expecting to need their bank accounts for medical costs. These savings convert into unplanned inheritances (De Nardi, French, and Jones, 2016; De Nardi, French, and Jones, 2010; Marshall et al., 2010; Suari-Andreu, Alessie, & Angelini, 2019; Venti & Wise, 2004). On this account, initial spending cuts are a predictable reaction to uncovered healthcare risks, potentially leaving retirees in a materially worse position.

That anticipation is not without reason. Retirees do, in fact, face significant costs for healthcare since most discover that their health insurance does not cover their prescription medication. The need to pay for medicines then forces spending cuts on other necessary items and propel some to seek low-return, low-risk, highly liquid investments that retirees can easily access to cover their bills. This slows the growth of future savings (Kotlikoff, 1986; Levin, 1995; Palumbo, 1999; Pang & Warshawsky, 2010). We can see the impact of this strategy when we consider how the opposite condition (adequate health insurance protection among Medicare eligible families) increases their allocation of savings—by 7.1% to 13% points—to more risk prone but presumably more lucrative assets (Goldman & Maestas, 2013).

It is unclear from the existing literature whether retirees can make substantial spending cuts without experiencing economic hardships and a decline in their standard of living. More research is necessary to understand what spending level workers need and expect to have in retirement.

Has the Retirement Outlook Gotten Worse?

The literature also shows increasing inequality in retirement income. Munnell et al. (2018) estimate that the share of working families at risk of an insecure retirement grew from 33% in 1983 to 53% in 2010 before declining to 50% in 2016. And Scholz et al. (2006) calculate that those born between 1931 and 1941 had only a 16% chance of falling below their optimal savings target in 1992, an estimate that grew to 25.9% by 2004 (Gale et al., 2009).

Moreover, studies broken down by age find that younger generations are less prepared for retirement than older cohorts (Newman, 2019). Butrica et al. (2012) project that 34% of those born between 1936 and 1945 could expect replacement rates of less than 75% and thus potentially face economic insecurity in retirement, compared to 39% for those born between 1946 and 1955, 41% for those born between 1956 and 1965 and 43% of those born between 1966 and 1975. These generational impacts reflect conditions in the labor market—from a rocky entry, to slow growth in wages, to lengthening spells of unemployment and the rise of the gig economy—that have impacted Generation X and everyone coming up behind them (Newman, 2019). Similarly, VanDerhei (2015) finds that savings shortfalls tend to be larger for younger cohorts, in large part because of higher future healthcare costs (VanDerhei, 2014).

Millennials, those born between 1981 and 1996, may disrupt this trend towards greater retirement income inequality. This generation seems to have put a greater emphasis on saving than previous cohorts since they started their careers during and immediately following the financial and economic crisis of 2007 to 2009. But only a minority of Millennials appear to participate in a retirement plan at work (Brown, 2018; Yao & Cheng, 2017) and have fewer assets and less wealth than GenXers at comparable times in their careers in 2001 (Kurz et al., 2018). In particular, they have had a more halting entry into the home ownership market (Newman, 2019). Researchers will need to analyze savings by age in the future to see whether the trend towards greater retirement income inequality has continued.

How Does Retirement Preparedness Differ by Race, Ethnicity, Gender, and Education?

Retirement wealth is unequally distributed by race and ethnicity, especially among groups that experience more income volatility. In 2016, 48% of Whites were at risk of an insecure retirement, compared to 54% for African Americans and 61% for Latinx (Munnell et al., 2018b). Those gaps widened from 1983 to 2016 (Munnell et al., 2018b). Edward Wolff (2015) also finds larger shares of non-White or Latinx households are unable to meet a replacement rate of 75% compared to Whites. Similarly, Butrica et al. (2012) project lower replacement rates and larger retirement income shortfalls for African Americans and Latinx than for Whites.

Researchers also consistently find larger shortfalls by gender. , for example, estimate that married women face the greatest risks with 45.6%, compared to, for example, 34.7% of widowed women. Married women face greater risks since they often outlive their husbands and use up much of the combined savings and thus face large shortfalls when they become widows. In a similar vein, Wolff (2015) projects that 59% of single women compared to 51% of single men will be unable to replace 75% of their preretirement income. And Butrica et al. (2012) project larger retirement shortfalls for women than for men.

Finally, some researchers provide estimates broken down by education. Wolff (2015), for instance, projects that 61% of those with less than 12 years of schooling could expect to fall short in retirement, compared to 43% of those with at least 16 years of education. Butrica et al. (2012) estimate the largest expected shortfalls for high school graduates and the smallest for college graduates.

Research using a living standard approach also finds large variations by race and gender. In 2016, 57% of women living alone potentially could not pay for basics, compared to 47% of men living alone and to only 27% of couples

(Mutchler et al., 2017a). Moreover, Hispanics had the highest chance of falling below the threshold with 74%, closely followed by African Americans with 67%, compared to 61% for Asian Americans and only 50% for Whites (Mutchler et al., 2017b). Similarly, Weller and Wolff (2005) find that while 23.2% of White near-retirees, those between 47 and 64 years old, could expect to have retirement incomes less than twice the poverty line, 56.6% of African American near-retirees could expect to fall short. Also, 33.3% of single men near retirement would have incomes lower than twice the poverty line, while 60.2% of single women would have lower incomes than that (Weller & Wolff, 2005).

Understanding retirement preparedness by race and ethnicity will require more research since very little information exists on the wealth distribution between Asian Americans and Whites and among Asian Americans. We have reason to believe this will be a problem worth studying because wealth tends to be more unequally distributed among Asian Americans than among Whites (Weller & Thompson, 2018). Moreover, non-White or Latinx population groups are growing faster than Whites, but most available data mask the social, cultural, historical and economic diversity within each group.

Researchers will also need to focus more attention on the gender dynamics of retirement preparedness, as do. The intersection between gender, marriage, divorce, and widowhood are especially important since those factors can pose particularly large economic risks for women (Couch et al., 2013; Weller & Tolson, 2017). Finally, while scholars often report estimates by education, the intersection between education and geography has gained increasing attention. Yet, very little research exists on the distribution of retirement wealth by region in isolation or in combination with education.

Is Income Inequality in Retirement Already Growing?
For the past three decades, we have seen a thunderous growth in income inequality. It stands to reason that this will impact retirees going forward. Bosworth, Burtless, and Zhang (2016) indeed find growing retirement income inequality, but this is largely an understudied area of research.

Figure 4.2 summarizes the share of income going to the top 10% of income earners among recent retirees (those who stopped working within the last 5 years and who are aged from 55 to 69 years). The share of income going to the top has gone up from 20.4% from 1989 to 1998 to 24.4% from 2010 to 2016 (Figure 4.2). At the same time, incomes of recent retirees appear to have stagnated for much of the past two decades (Gillers et al., 2018). In fact, Katherine Newman (2019) argues that retirement income inequality has widened to a point, where families, who once were securely middle class now face financial struggles in their retirement.

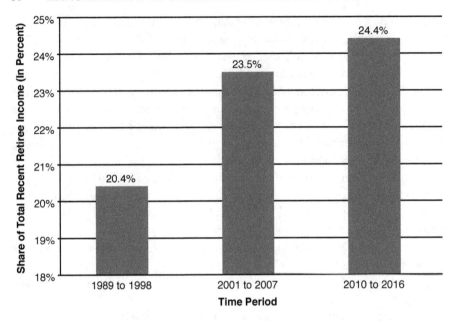

FIGURE 4.2 Share of income received by top 10% of those retired within last 5 years aged 55 to 69 years, by time period.

Analyzing these trends poses particular challenges for researchers. Projections of retirement preparedness assume a uniform retirement age across all households. Yet, households' retirement decisions will in part be determined by the need to work longer to compensate for low savings and the ability to work longer due to emerging health issues, especially among households with low wealth (Bosworth et al., 2016). Untangling the resulting heterogeneity in retirement incomes that follows from the combination of wealth, labor force participation, and health status will require further, detailed analyses.

How Do Private Retirement Savings Contribute to Retirement Inequality?

Workers who save for their retirement typically do so with the aid of a DB pension or a DC retirement account. The share of workers saving outside of the employer–employee relationship with an Individual Retirement Account (IRA) is very small (Chen & Munnell, 2017; Holden & Schrass, 2016). Among employment-based retirement plans, DC accounts have largely taken the place of DB pensions. Defined contributions require workers to make all of the relevant decisions, each of which exposes them to the chance of losing substantial shares of their savings. These decisions include choosing to participate in a retirement plan in the first place, deciding on how much and when to contribute, how to invest the money and when and how much to withdraw before and then during retirement.

These complexities lead many workers to refrain from participating in an employer-sponsored retirement plan altogether, even when one is available. The Bureau of Labor Statistics (n.d.) reports that only 75% of the workers that had access to a DC plan in 2018 actually participated in it. Some workers may not be eligible for a DC plan because they work too few hours or haven't worked in that establishment long enough (Pew Charitable Trusts, 2017). Often workers are ineligible because they work too few or irregular hours, a key contributor to income volatility, which then spills over into retirement wealth. Other workers do not think that they have the disposable income to save for retirement (Pew Charitable Trusts, 2017). Again, workers tend to cite unpredictable schedules and earnings as a key obstacle to saving (Aspen Institute, 2019), so that the growth of income volatility could contribute to rising wealth inequality. Many find it hard to get over inertia (Thaler & Benartzi, 2004). This reticence has consequences: Workers will lose out on the value of an employer match for their savings and they will not reap any potential tax benefits from saving in a DC account such as a 401(k) or 403(b) (Brady, 2012; Ghilarducci & Weller, 2015).

To increase retirement savings plan participation, more and more employers have created "opt out" options, whereby workers are automatically enrolled in a 401(k) type plan at work, but can decline to participate. Inspired by observations in behavioral economics, this approach lowers the barriers to participation by taking decision-making out of the picture (Choi et al., 2004; Madrian & Shea, 2001). Perhaps employers recognize this psychological reality, since 46% of employers offered automatic enrollment features in 2017, up from just 1% in 2003 (Clark, Utkus, & Young, 2015). Accordingly, thousands of workers have no "opt out" pathway and must either engage on their own or lose.

Workers who participate in a DC plan still need to decide how much and when to contribute. They could decide, for instance, to contribute very little and only do so on an irregular basis. Earnings volatility and the associated lack of predictability keeps contributions low (Ghilarducci et al., 2018), so that greater volatility widens retirement wealth inequality. Employees also positively respond to employer match rates (Duflo et al., 2006). The effectiveness of these matches can be limited by employee inertia (Choi et al., 2011).

Once workers decide to save for retirement, they need to pick investments, which is a very complex decision that few are prepared to make. Instead, many workers will use heuristics when making investment decisions (Benartzi & Thaler, 2007; Frydman & Camerer, 2016) which could result in investing too much money in employer stock (Benartzi, 2001; Poterba, 2003), putting too much or too little money in stocks in general (Benartzi & Thaler, 2001, 2007), and buying high, while selling low (Frydman & Camerer, 2016). These financial risks could generate less wealth and contribute to more inequality, since those with more resources also get more professional advice and are likely more familiar with the logic of investing.

Theoretically workers should rebalance their investments by selling stocks and buying more bonds to reap the maximum value on their investments, but in practice very few actually do (Mitchell, Mottola, Utkus, & Yamaguchi, 2008). Without rebalancing, workers end up with more risk than they are comfortable with. They lose more of their savings than they are willing to tolerate, which could lead them to move more money to liquid, low-risk investments as a response.

Workers saving with a DC account face hard-to-avoid market risks. Both stock prices and bond market interest rates can remain well below average often for decades. Long periods of an underperforming stock market tend to be followed by a period of above-average returns (Campbell & Shiller, 1998, 2001). Workers typically do not have the time to wait decades until stock and bond markets return to average or above-average levels and help them generate more savings. Depending on when they start to save, they could end up with relatively low savings balances (Shiller, 2005; Weller, 2019).

Some households are better positioned than others to handle the risks associated with DC accounts. Wealthier households can absorb a larger drop in their retirement savings due to poor decisions or a market downturn than less wealthy ones can. Wealth is increasingly concentrated among higher-income and White households. But, those are also the households least likely to experience income volatility during their working lives and thus least likely to need to rely on their savings in an emergency.

Workers with DB pensions typically do not face any of these risks. These employees qualify for a DB pension and participate automatically. There is generally no discretion in how much to contribute and all DB pensions offer an annuity options. Because DB plans protect workers from many risks, the switch to DC accounts over the past three decades has gone along with growing wealth inequality among those workers who are covered by a retirement plan at work.

Figure 4.3 summarizes the distribution of wealth among preretired households by retirement plan type from 2010 to 2016, based on Federal Reserve data (Board of Governors, Federal Reserve System, 2019; Sabelhaus & Henriques, 2019). In each case, the distribution is calculated separately for households with only DC accounts, for those with a DB pension and for those with neither a DC account nor a DB pension. DC accounts include 401(k) type accounts as well as IRAs, which are mainly funds rolled over from 401(k)s from prior jobs.

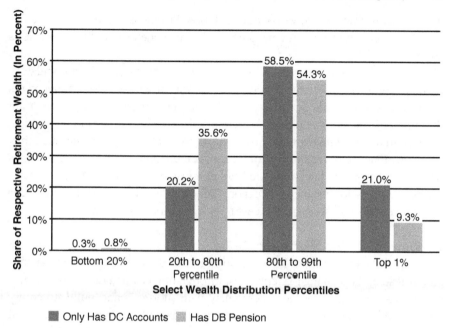

FIGURE 4.3 Distribution of retirement wealth by type of retirement benefit from 2010 to 2016.

Importantly, the rise in wealth and retirement income inequality associated with changing retirement benefits applies only to a subset of the population. Most Asian Americans and Latinx workers are not covered by a retirement plan at work and only half of African Americans were in 2014, compared to 57% of Whites (Harvey, 2017). Lower-income workers also have less access to employment-based retirement plans than higher-income ones (Joint Committee on Taxation, U.S. Congress, 2019; Pew Charitable Trusts, 2017). The bigger retirement income inequality is the difference between those who have a retirement plan and those who do not. Many of the risks of DC accounts as well as the shortcomings of the voluntary retirement savings system have been studied in detail.

More research will be needed to address the feasibility and effectiveness of proposed solutions to minimize the risks of DC accounts, especially for workers that face a large chance of income volatility in their daily lives. Policy makers at the federal and state levels, for instance, have proposed to create retirement savings options, supported by government administrations to ensure low-cost, low-risk investments. These proposals would require employers above a certain size to offer all employees a retirement plan at work or offer payroll deduction into an IRA if there is no employer-sponsored retirement plan. The money would be invested in low-cost, low-risk mutual funds. Proposals include the option to withdraw some money in an emergency and some benefits could be available as annuities.

These proposals raise several key research questions. First, can mandatory participation increase savings among workers with irregular work arrangements such as part-time workers and workers in the gig economy? Second, what are the limits of opt out savings? It is possible that the workers most in need of more retirement savings are also the ones most likely to opt out because they need the money to cover short-term income fluctuations. Third, can plan designs better protect against hard-to-avoid market and longevity risks? As a few state-sponsored plans, for instance, in Oregon, California, and Illinois are getting under way, researchers will soon have access to new data to consider these issues.

Is Homeownership Worth the Risks?

Many workers with volatile incomes do not have dedicated retirement savings and instead end up saving for retirement through homeownership. This is a form of forced savings since homeowners repay their mortgage and build up equity (Herbert et al., 2013). Homeownership thus partially overcomes behavioral obstacles to saving such as inertia, especially among families that experience volatile incomes. Homeownership also provides a stream of in-kind income in retirement as most people plan on staying in their house (Society of Actuaries, 2018) and end up doing so in retirement (Venti & Wise, 2004). Relatedly, housing is a partial insurance against longevity risk (Poterba et al., 2011), so that housing assets can generate relatively more value for retirees than other nonannuitized assets.

Homeownership allows generations—adult children, parents, and grandparents—to support each other, for instance, by temporarily living under the same roof. Katherine Newman's research on "accordion families" in the United States, Western Europe, and Japan, make it clear that countries with high levels of home ownership and weak welfare states are seeing an increase in the length of time adult children live with their parents. On the plus side, these intergenerational living arrangements enable families to spread the risks of income volatility between different generations. On the minus side, these same arrangements are leading to marriages foregone and low fertility, with significant implications for economic growth (Newman, 2012).

Homeownership carries positive externalities that offer additional benefits to homeowners because it is geographically specific (Coulson, 2002). Owners tend to spend more on their own house than is the case for renters (Crone, 2006; DiPasquale and Glaeser, 1999; Galster, 1983; Harding et al., 2000). Owner-occupied housing holds value longer than rental properties (Shilling et al., 1991).

And neighborhoods with greater homeownership rates have better educational outcomes (Green & White, 1997; Haurin et al., 2002; Rohe & Lindblad, 2013), more recreational amenities, and more civic engagement (Rohe & Lindblad, 2013). All of these factors boost housing wealth and could in part address savings shortfalls for families with volatile incomes.

Homeownership, though, raises costs for retirees since they have to maintain their house. Moreover, they cannot easily convert a house into cash (Ellis et al., 2014; Sinai & Souleles, 2007) when they need to pay for other things such as medical care (De Nardi, et al., 2016, 2010; Marshall et al., 2010). To address these costs, retirees often spend less and build up savings in retirement (De Nardi et al., 2016; Suari-Andreu et al., 2019; Venti & Wise, 2004). They end up spending too little on other things such as food and healthcare to self-insure against the risks associated with homeownership, since they have fewer liquid savings than renters to pay for those expenses (Nakajima & Telyukova, 2012).

These competing benefits and risks translate into a rate of return for housing investments that are greater than for treasuries but below that of stocks (Jud & Winkler, 2005). Yet, the risks of housing investment is greater than that of either or treasuries (Jud & Winkler, 2005). Some researchers then conclude that homeownership does not in fact increase savings (Krumm & Kelly, 1989) and that low-income households do not build wealth faster as homeowners than renters (Wainer & Zabel, 2019). Because the risks are unevenly distributed by income and possibly by income volatility, though, housing contributes to increasing wealth inequality over time.

Researchers will need to consider several broad questions related to housing as a source of retirement income in the context of the link between income volatility and retirement savings. First, under what circumstances do families experiencing income volatility tolerate the risks associated with homeownership? It may be particularly beneficial for these homeowners to help them build savings outside of their house. It could also include shared equity purchases that spread the risks and benefits of homeownership between lower-income purchasers and lenders. In addition, how do homeowners fare with their retirement savings compared to renters? Who faces greater economic risks with their tenure choice, especially after the housing market crash after 2007?

Do Family Caregivers Save Less For Retirement?
In 2016, approximately 40 million people in the United States were providing unpaid care to adults (Rainville et al., 2016). More than half of all caregivers are responsible for parents and spouses (Collinson & De La Torre, 2017). Women are more likely to be unpaid caregivers which exacerbates the existing gender

wealth gap (Arano, Parker, & Terry, 2010; Butrica et al., 2012; Deere & Doss, 2006; Glass & Kilpatrick, 1998; Sunden & Surette, 1998; Wolff, 2017). Family caregiving increases what is already widespread economic insecurity among older women, in particular, and minority women especially (Glass & Kilpatrick, 1998; Harris & Werman, 2014; Minkler & Stone, 1985; Newman, 2003; Warlick, 1985).

Median 401(k) balances have widened by gender as Figure 4.4 shows. This growing wealth gap follows from increasing differences in experiences at work related to caregiving (Weller & Tolson, 2017). People need to have a job to qualify for a 401(k) plan and most unpaid family caregivers still work for pay in their noncaregiving job (Collinson & De La Torre, 2017; National Alliance of Caregivers and AARP Public Policy Institute, 2015). Unpaid caregiving adversely impacts labor market outcomes—earnings, hours, and job stability— as well as health (Newman 2003; Pinquart & Sorensen, 2003a, 2003b; Pinquart & Sorensen, 2006; 2007). These factors impact savings and retirement wealth among caregivers (Bogan & Fertig, 2018; Weller & Tolson, 2017). The consequences of these gender inequalities are more serious for women (Weller & Thompson, 2018; Weller & Tolson, 2017) since they are more likely to be caregivers and often provide more intensive care than men do (NAC & AARP, 2015; Pavalko & Artis, 1997).

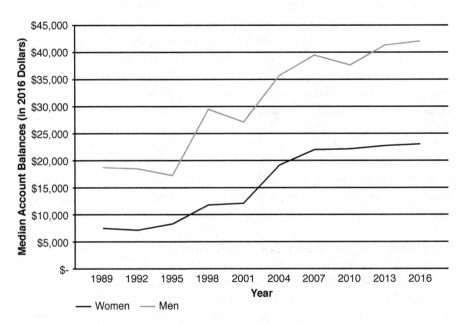

FIGURE 4.4 Median real retirement savings balances by gender from 1989 to 2016.

Saving for one's own retirement critically depends on employment. Higher earnings allow households to save more, not just because they can more easily pay their bills. The tax code also incentivizes more savings for higher earners. Having a job increases the likelihood of work-based retirement benefits, a crucial means of growing assets. Finally, stable employment allows people to save and invest over longer periods of time, which translates into higher returns and more savings, as we discussed previously.

There is limited evidence on the link between caregiving and wealth and nothing that links income volatility among caregivers to savings. Weller and Tolson (2017) show that caregivers—including both child and adult care—are less likely to have a 401(k) plan, especially among single women. The Government Accountability Office (GAO, 2019) finds that spousal caregiving correlates with lower retirement savings and less wealth near retirement, for instance. Van Houtven et al. (2010), however, find no link between parental caregiving and Social Security wealth.

It is alternatively possible that caregivers anticipated that they will care for a family member and saved more to prepare for this eventuality. There is evidence that some caregivers at least partially base their decision of whether or not to become caregivers on their own finances, although this tends to be true only of a minority. If caregivers indeed prepare for their own future, their total wealth should be higher or comparable to that of noncaregivers as they near retirement. The existing research only provides very limited evidence on the link between unpaid care and wealth. As adult caregiving increases in an aging society, more research will need to consider the link between the economic instability that results from family care, on the one hand, and savings, on the other. Researchers will need to distinguish between the effects of different types of caregiving, for instance, for parents, spouses and disabled family members. They will also need to consider whether caregivers consider their own finances in deciding to care for somebody else and thus make financial plans accordingly. And they will look at the longer-term effects of caregiving to see whether past caregivers may be able to recover some of the potential losses. In short, our understanding of the whole caregiving "nexus" needs to broaden out from a traditional emphasis on individuals and earnings/savings to a more holistic intergenerational understanding.

Do Healthcare and Education Costs Stand in the Way of More Retirement Savings?

Families face increasing costs for key items such as healthcare and education that exacerbate the effects of low incomes, declining income mobility, and rising income volatility. All of these factors make it harder for families to save. While income inequality has widened, mobility has fallen and volatility has increased. The costs of education and student loans, though, have increased, which means households must save more to be well prepared for these costs. Families end up going deeper into debt to pay for their own and for their children's education and to cover unexpected healthcare expenses. The costs of student loans and medical debt are unequally distributed; both amplify wealth inequality.

Families increasingly borrow for their own education and that of their children (Federal Reserve Bank of New York [FRBNY], 2019). Student loans have particularly increased among younger households after the Great Recession ended since colleges and universities increased their tuition rates (Bleemer, Brown, Lee, Strair, & Van der Klaauw, 2017). And student loans are more widespread among African American students and other families of color than among Whites (Espinosa et al., 2019; Huelsman, 2015). Yet people of color with student loans earn less than Whites when they graduate, resulting in an ever widening student loan difference by race (Addo, Houle, & Simon, 2016; Grinstein-Weiss et al., 2016; Scott-Clayton & Li, 2016). This is partly a reflection of the kinds of institutions that student loan recipients attend; a higher proportion of African Americans attend for-profit colleges which typically increase loan burdens, have high dropout rates, and see lower earnings among graduates than public sector or nonprofit institutions.

More African American than White families also owe student debt for students who never graduated (Goldrick-Rab et al., 2014; Huelsman, 2015). Earnings increases, though, are smaller for people with only some college education who didn't graduate than for those who did. This debt further widens the racial wealth gap which is not limited to younger households, but also impacts older ones since many student loans are disproportionately owed by African American parents (Walsemann & Ailshire, 2016). Not surprisingly, a growing share of retirees still owe student loans, especially for their grandchildren (for whom they have cosigned).

Student debt consequently exacerbates retirement wealth inequality. Almost three quarters of households with student loans have not saved for retirement (Elliott & Lewis, 2015). Student loan borrowers also appear more likely to stop saving for retirement or to withdraw their retirement savings when the economy enters a recession and income volatility increases (Elliott et al., 2013). And those who owe student loans are more likely to experience financial vulnerabilities than those without them (Despard et al., 2016). The risk of these financial difficulties is unevenly distributed as Marshall Steinbaum and Kavya Vaghul (2016) find. Student loan delinquencies are concentrated among Latinx and African American borrowers using credit reporting data by zip code. Student loan debt thus likely magnifies the link between income volatility and wealth inequality.

Healthcare costs also tighten the link between income volatility and wealth inequality. Many people who suffer from chronic health conditions borrow to pay for their healthcare, especially when they have no health insurance or their insurance covers only part of their health expenses (Doty et al., 2005; Richard et al., 2018; Zeldin & Rukovina, 2008). This medical debt increases the risk of bankruptcy (Himmelstein et al., 2009, 2005; Seifert & Rukavina, 2006; Warren & Warren, 2004). Medical-debt–related bankruptcies reduce wealth since most families with medical debt who filed for bankruptcy first exhausted other savings and many went deeper into other debt (Seifert & Rukavina, 2006). Moreover, people with medical debt appear to seek less medical care (Choi, 2018; Kalousova & Burgard, 2013). The lack of care can make it harder for people to get back to their jobs and build savings. At the same time, indebtedness, including medical debt, causes stress and worsens health outcomes (Turunen & Hiilamo, 2014). Poor health raises the chance of more debt, which in turn increases the chance of poor health. This vicious cycle lowers wealth for affected households by both reducing their savings and reducing their earnings potential.

The link between student loans and medical debt, on the one hand, and retirement preparedness on the other will require researchers' further attention since both forms of debt have grown significantly in recent decades despite the advent of the Affordable Care Act in 2009. The key challenge for researchers will be to better understand the causality between student loans and wealth near and in retirement. This will require disentangling the influences of intermediating factors such as students' own earnings as well as their parents' finances on this connection.

With respect to medical debt, it will be critical to better understand how the Affordable Care Act has impacted medical debt and its distribution between varying population groups. One key issue will be to see whether better insurance coverage has resulted in more equitable healthcare access and fewer inequities in health outcomes by income and race, for example. More health insurance under the Affordable Care Act appears to have initially reduced medical debt, but those improvements eventually stalled (Collins et al., 2019). Researchers interested in the link between medical debt and retirement inequality will need to further analyze the reasons for the slowdown as well as the distributional aspects by income, age and race of medical debt changes associated with more health insurance coverage.

CONCLUSION

Retirement wealth inequality has increased for three decades. Increasingly, income inequality among recent retirees has gone up, too. This growth follows from decades of increasing inequality and falling mobility as well as growing income volatility.

Income volatility and key economic risks related to this uncertainty are understudied contributors to a lack of savings among younger cohorts, women, and communities of color. We summarize the evidence to show that income volatility contributes to fewer retirement savings. Moreover, income volatility appears to be linked to other economic risk factors that make it harder for people to save for their future. These risk factors include the use of retirement savings accounts, homeownership, student loans, and medical debt.

We point to a number of open research questions related to income volatility and its connection to retirement wealth inequality. Answering these questions could provide better insights on the distribution of the risks associated with this instability. These answers will give policy makers a sense of the target audiences if they want to create more economic stability prior to retirement. In addition, answering these open research questions could also offer evidence on the causal mechanisms by which more income volatility lowers retirement savings. A better understanding of the link between income volatility and its associated factors, on the one hand, and wealth inequality, on the other hand, would identify pathways for new policy interventions to help people save more for their retirement.

NOTES

1. This threshold is less than 100% as retirees need less income than workers since they no longer need to save for retirement and have fewer work-related expenses.
2. Browning & Lusardi (1996) provide a summary of the neoclassical literature on consumption and saving that links current and future consumption through current savings.
3. Most estimates use spending rather than consumption as the key metric. Many lower-income retirees will likely be able to consume more than they can spend since they can access public assistance programs. Scholz et al. (2006) include the likelihood of receiving public assistance in their estimates based on eligibility rules, take up rates and funding for public programs. This reduces the share of retirees ill prepared for retirement at the lower end of the income spectrum, but this is an inherently problematic assumption since eligibility, take up, and funding can unpredictably and quickly change. We thus use future spending rather than consumption in much of our review.

4. Differences in estimated retirement preparedness also result from separate target replacement rates. The target replacement rate implied by financial service industry standards tend to be well above 80% of preretirement income, while researchers often use replacement rates around 70% (Biggs & Springstead, 2008). Reaching lower target replacement rates will require less savings and thus show smaller shortfalls.

REFERENCES

Addo, F. R., Houle, J. N., & Simon, D. (2016). Young, black, and (still) in the red: Parental wealth, race, and student loan debt. *Race and Social Problems*, 8(1), 64–76. https://doi.org/10.1007/s12552-016-9162-0

Aguiar, M., & Hurst, E. (2005). Consumption versus expenditure. *Journal of political Economy*, 113(5), 919–948. https://doi.org/10.1086/491590

Aguiar, M., & Hurst, E. (2013). Deconstructing life cycle expenditure. *Journal of Political Economy*, 121(3), 437–492. https://doi.org/10.1086/670740

Aguila, E., Attanasio, O., & Meghir, C. (2011). Changes in consumption at retirement: Evidence from panel data. *Review of Economics and Statistics*, 93(3), 1094–1099.

Ameriks, J., & Utkus, S. P. (2006). *Vanguard retirement outlook 2006*. Vanguard Center for Retirement Research. King of Prussia, PA: Vanguard.

Arano, K., Parker, C., & Terry, R. (2010). Gender based risk aversion and retirement asset allocation. *Economic Inquiry*, 48(1), 147–155. https://doi.org/10.1111/j.1465-7295.2008.00201.x

Aspen Institute. (2019). *Short-term financial stability: A foundation for security and well-being*. Washington, DC: Aspen Institute. Consumer Insight Collaborative.

Banks, J., Blundell, R., & Tanner, S. (1998). Is there a retirement-savings puzzle? *American Economic Review*, 769–788.

Benartzi, S. (2001). Excessive extrapolation and the allocation of 401 (k) accounts to company stock. *The Journal of Finance*, 56(5), 1747–1764. https://doi.org/10.1111/0022-1082.00388

Benartzi, S., & Thaler, R. H. (2001). Naive diversification strategies in defined contribution saving plans. *American Economic Review*, 91(1), 79–98. https://doi.org/10.1257/aer.91.1.79

Benartzi, S., & Thaler, R. H. (2007). Heuristics and biases in retirement savings behavior. *Journal of Economic Perspectives*, 21(3), 81–104. https://doi.org/10.1257/jep.21.3.81

Benito, A. (2006). Does job insecurity affect household consumption? *Oxford Economic Papers*, 58(1), 157–181. https://doi.org/10.1093/oep/gpi041

Bernheim, B. D. (1997). The adequacy of personal retirement saving: Issues and options. In D. Wise (Ed.), *Facing the age wave* (pp. 30–56). Palo Alto, CA: Hoover Institute Press.

Bernheim, B. D., Skinner, J., & Weinberg, S. (2001). What accounts for the variation in retirement wealth among US households? *American Economic Review, 91*(4), 832–857. https://doi.org/10.1257/aer.91.4.832

Biggs, A. G., & Springstead, G. R. (2008). Alternate measures of replacement rates for social security benefits and retirement income. *Social Security Bulletin, 68,* 1.

Blanchett, D. (2013). *Estimating the true cost of retirement.* Chicago, IL: Morningstar.

Bleemer, Z., Brown, M., Lee, D., Strair, K., & Van der Klaauw, W. (2017). *Echoes of rising tuition in students' borrowing, educational attainment, and homeownership in post-recession America.* Staff Report No. 820. New York, NY: Federal Reserve Bank of New York.

Board of Governors, Federal Reserve System. (2014). *Report on the economic well-being of U.S. Households in 2013.* Washington, DC: Fed.

Board of Governors, Federal Reserve System. (2019). *Survey of consumer finances, various years.* Washington, DC: Fed.

Bogan, V., & Fertig, A. (2018). Mental health and retirement savings: Confounding issues with compounding interest. *Health Economics, 27,* 404–425. https://doi.org/10.1002/hec.3579

Boskin, M. J., & Shoven, J. B. (1984). Concepts and measures of earnings replacement during retirement. In Z. Bodie, J. B. Shoven, & D. A. Wise, *Issues in pension economics* (pp. 113–141). Chicago, IL: University of Chicago Press.

Bosworth, B., Burtless, G., & Zhang, K. (2016). *Later retirement, inequality in old age, and the growing gap in longevity between rich and poor.* Washington, DC: Brookings Institution.

Brady, P. J. (2012). *The tax benefits and revenue costs of tax deferral.* Investment Company Institute White Paper. Washington, DC: Investment Company Institute.

Brown, J. E. (2018). *Millennials and retirement: Already falling short.* NIRS Report. Washington, DC: National Institute for Retirement Security.

Browning, M., & Lusardi, A. (1996). Household saving: Micro theories and micro facts. *Journal of Economic literature, 34*(4), 1797–1855.

Bureau of Labor Statistics. (n.d.). *Employee benefits survey. Table 1: Retirement benefits: Access, participation, and take-up rates, civilian workers.* Washington, DC: Author. Retrieved from https://www.bls.gov/news.release/ebs2.t01.htm

Butrica, B. A., Smith, K. E., & Iams, H. M. (2012). This is not your parents' retirement: Comparing retirement income across generations. *Social Security Bulletin, 72,* 37.

Cagetti, M. (2003). Wealth accumulation over the life cycle and precautionary savings. *Journal of Business & Economic Statistics, 21*(3), 339–353. https://doi.org/10.1198/073500103288619007

Campbell, J. Y., & Shiller, R. J. (1998). Valuation ratios and the long-run stock market outlook. *The Journal of Portfolio Management, 24*(2), 11–26. https://doi.org/10.3905/jpm.24.2.11

Campbell, J. Y., & Shiller, R. J. (2001). *Valuation ratios and the long-run stock market outlook: An update* (No. w8221). Cambridge, MA: National Bureau of Economic Research.

Carroll, C. D., & Samwick, A. A. (1998). How important is precautionary saving? *Review of Economics and Statistics, 80*(3), 410–419. https://doi.org/10.1162/003465398557645

Center for Social and Demographic Research on Aging, University of Massachusetts Boston and Gerontology Institute, University of Massachusetts Boston. (2017). *The National Elder Economic Security Standard™ Index: Methodology overview.* Center for Social and Demographic Research on Aging publications. Boston, MA: University of Massachusetts Boston.

Chen, A., & Munnell, A. H. (2017). *Who contributes to individual retirement accounts* (No. ib2017-8). Issue in Brief, 17-8. Boston, MA: Center for Retirement Research, Boston College.

Chetty, R. (2016, Fall). *Improving opportunities for economic mobility: New evidence and policy lessons.* St. Louis, MO: Federal Reserve Bank of St. Louis.

Chetty, R., Grusky, D., Hell, M., Hendren, N., Manduca, R., & Narang, J. (2017). The fading American dream: Trends in absolute income mobility since 1940. *Science, 356*(6336), 398–406. https://doi.org/10.1126/science.aal4617

Chetty, R., Hendren, N., Kline, C. B., Saez, D. (2014). Active vs. passive decisions and crowd-out in retirement savings accounts: Evidence from Denmark. *The Quarterly Journal of Economics, 129*(3), 1141–1219. https://doi.org/10.1093/qje/qju013

Chetty, R., Hendren, N., Kline, P., & Saez, E. (2014). Where is the land of opportunity? The geography of intergenerational mobility in the United States. *The Quarterly Journal of Economics, 129*(4), 1553–1623. https://doi.org/10.1093/qje/qju022

Choi, J. J., Laibson, D. I., & Madrian, B. C. (2004). *Plan design and 401 (k) savings outcomes* (No. w10486). Cambridge, MA: National Bureau of Economic Research.

Choi, J. J., Laibson, D. I., & Madrian, B. C. (2011). $100 Bills on the sidewalk: Suboptimal investment in 401(k) plans. *Review of Economics and Statistics, 93*(3), 748–763.

Choi, S. (2018). Experiencing financial hardship associated with medical bills and its effects on health care behavior: A 2-year panel study. *Health Education & Behavior, 45*(4), 616–624. https://doi.org/10.1177/1090198117739671

Clark, J. W., Utkus, S. P., & Young, J. A. (2015). *Automatic enrollment: The power of the default.* Valley Forge. PA: Vanguard.

Collins, S. R., Bhupal, H. K., & Doty, M. M. (2019). Health insurance coverage eight years after the ACA. *Commonwealth Fund, 7,* 1–28.

Collinson, C., & De La Torre, H. (2017). The many faces of caregivers: A close-up look at caregiving and its impacts. *Transamerica Institute,* pp. 1–299.

Couch, K. A., Tamborini, C. R., Reznik, G. L., & Phillips, J. W. (2013). Divorce, women's earnings, and retirement over the life course. In K. Couch, M. C. Daly, & J. Zissimopoulos (Eds.), *Lifecycle events and their consequences: Job loss, family change, and declines in health* (pp. 133–157, chap. 8). Palo Alto, CA: Stanford University Press.

Coulson, N. E. (2002). Housing policy and the social benefits of homeownership. *Business Review, 2,* 7–16.

Crone, T. M. (2006). *Capitalization of the quality of local public schools: What do home buyers value?* (FRPHL Working Paper No. 06-15). Philadelphia, PA: Federal Reserve Bank of Philadelphia.

Dahl, M. W., DeLeire, T. C., & Schwabish, J. A. (2007). *Trends in earnings variability over the past 20 years.* Congress of the United States, Congressional Budget Office. Washington, DC: Congressional Budget Office.

Deere, C. D., & Doss, C. R. (2006). The gender asset gap: What do we know and why does it matter? *Feminist Economics, 12*(1–2), 1–50. https://doi.org/10.1080/13545700500508056

De Nardi., M, French., E, & Jones, J. B. (2010). Why do the elderly save? The role of medical expenses. *Journal of Political Economy, 118*(1), 39–75. https://doi.org/10.1086/651674

De Nardi., M, French., E, & Jones, J. B. (2016). Savings after retirement: A survey. *Annual Review of Economics, 8,* 177–204.

Despard, M. R., Perantie, D., Taylor, S., Grinstein-Weiss, M., Friedline, T., & Raghavan, R. (2016). Student debt and hardship: Evidence from a large sample of low- and moderate-income households. *Children and Youth Services Review, 70,* 8–18. https://doi.org/10.1016/j.childyouth.2016.09.001

DiPasquale, D., & Glaeser, E. L. (1999). Incentives and social capital: Are homeowners better citizens? *Journal of Urban Economics, 45*(2), 354–384. https://doi.org/10.1006/juec.1998.2098

Doty, M. M., Edwards, J. N., & Holmgren, A. L. (2005). *Seeing red: Americans driven into debt by medical bills.* New York, NY: The Commonwealth Fund.

Duflo, E., Gale, W., Liebman, J., Orszag, P., & Saez, E. (2006). Saving incentives for low-and middle-income families: Evidence from a field experiment with H&R Block. *The Quarterly Journal of Economics, 121*(4), 1311–1346. https://doi.org/10.1162/qjec.121.4.1311

Dynan, K., Elmendorf, D., & Sichel, D. (2012). The evolution of household income volatility. *The BE Journal of Economic Analysis & Policy, 12*(2), 1–42. https://doi.org/10.1515/1935-1682.3347

Elliott, W., Grinstein-Weiss, M., & Nam, I. (2013). *Student debt and declining retirement savings* (CSD Working Paper 13–34). St. Louis, MO: Center for Social Development, Washington University.

Elliott, W., & Lewis, M. (2015). Student debt effects on financial well-being: Research and policy implications. *Journal of Economic Surveys, 29*(4), 614–636. https://doi.org/10.1111/joes.12124

Ellis, C. D., Munnell, A. H., & Eschtruth, A. D. (2014). *Falling short: The coming retirement crisis and what to do about it.* New York, NY: Oxford University Press.

Engen, E. M., Gale, W. G., & Uccello, C. E. (2005). Lifetime earnings, Social Security benefits, and the adequacy of retirement wealth accumulation. *Social Security Bulletin,*
66, 38. https://doi.org/10.2139/ssrn.546243

Engen, E. M., Gale, W. G., Uccello, C. E., Carroll, C. D., & Laibson, D. I. (1999). The
adequacy of household saving. *Brookings Papers on Economic Activity, 1999*(2), 65–
187. https://doi.org/10.2307/2534679

Espinosa, L. L., Turk, J. M., Taylor, M., & Chessman, H. M. (2019). *Race and eth-*
nicity in higher education: A status report. Washington, DC: American Council on
Education.

Federal Reserve Bank of New York, Center for Microeconomic Data. (2019). *Household*
debt and credit report, First Quarter 2019. New York, NY: Author.

Frydman, C., & Camerer, C. F. (2016). The psychology and neuroscience of financial decision making. *Trends in Cognitive Sciences, 20*(9), 661–675. https://doi.org/
10.1016/j.tics.2016.07.003

Gale, W., Scholz, J. K., & Seshadri, A. (2009). *Are all Americans saving 'optimally' for retire-*
ment? Michigan Retirement Research Center Working Paper wp189. Ann Arbor,
MI: Michigan Retirement Research Center, University of Michigan.

Galster, G. C. (1983). Empirical evidence on cross-tenure differences in home maintenance and conditions. *Land Economics, 59*(1), 107–113.

Ghilarducci, T., Saad-Lessler, J., & Reznik, G. (2018). Earnings volatility and 401
(k) contributions. *Journal of Pension Economics & Finance, 17*(4), 554–575.
https://doi.org/10.1017/S1474747217000178

Ghilarducci, T., & Weller, C. E. (2015). *The inefficiencies of existing retirement savings incen-*
tives. (No. 2015-02). Schwartz Center for Economic Policy Analysis (SCEPA), The
New School.

Gillers, H., Tergesen, A., & Scism, L. (2018). A Generation of Americans is entering old age the least prepared in decades. *The Wall Street Journal.* Retrieved
from https://www.wsj.com/articles/a-generation-of-americans-is-entering-old-age-
the-least-prepared-in-decades-1529676033

Glass, Jr., C, J., & Kilpatrick, B. B. (1998). Financial planning for retirement: An imper-
ative for baby boomer women. *Educational Gerontology: An International Quarterly,*
24(6), 595–617. https://doi.org/10.1080/0360127980240606

Golden, L. (2015). Irregular work scheduling and its consequences. *Economic Policy Insti-*
tute Briefing Paper, (394), 1–44.

Goldman, D., & Maestas, N. (2013). Medical expenditure risk and household portfolio choice. *Journal of Applied Econometrics, 28*(4), 527–550. https://doi.org/
10.1002/jae.2278

Goldrick-Rab, S., Kelchen, R., & Houle, J. (2014). The color of student debt: Implications
of federal loan program reforms for black students and historically black colleges
and universities (pp. 1–44) Madison, WI: Wisconsin HOPE Lab.

Gollier, C., & Pratt, J. W. (1996). Risk vulnerability and the tempering effect of background risk. *Econometrica: Journal of the Econometric Society, 64*(5), 1109–1123. https://doi.org/10.2307/2171958

Gonyea, J. G. (2007). Improving the retirement prospects of lower-wage workers in a defined-contribution world. *Families in Society, 88*(3), 453–462.

Gottschalk, P., Moffitt, R., Katz, L. F., & Dickens, W. T. (1994). The growth of earnings instability in the US labor market. *Brookings Papers on Economic Activity, 1994*(2), 217–272. https://doi.org/10.2307/2534657

Gourinchas, P. O., & Parker, J. A. (2001). The empirical importance of precautionary saving. *American Economic Review, 91*(2), 406–412. https://doi.org/10.1257/aer.91.2.406

Government Accountability Office. (2019). *Retirement security: Income and wealth disparities continue through old age.* GAO Report No. GAO-19-587. Washington, DC: GAO.

Green, R. K., & White, M. J. (1997). Measuring the benefits of homeowning: Effects on children. *Journal of Urban Economics, 41*(3), 441–461.

Grinstein-Weiss, M., Perantie, D. C., Taylor, S. H., Guo, S., & Raghavan, R. (2016). Racial disparities in education debt burden among low-and moderate-income households. *Children and Youth Services Review, 65*, 166–174. https://doi.org/10.1016/j.childyouth.2016.04.010

Guiso, L., Jappelli, T., & Terlizzese, D. (1992). Earnings uncertainty and precautionary saving. *Journal of Monetary Economics, 30*(2), 307–337. https://doi.org/10.1016/0304-3932(92)90064-9

Guiso, L., Jappelli, T., & Terlizzese, D. (1996). Income risk, borrowing constraints, and portfolio choice. *The American Economic Review, 86*(1), 158–172.

Gustman, A. L., & Steinmeier, T. L. (1999, June). Effects of pensions on savings: Analysis with data from the Health and Retirement Study. *Carnegie-Rochester Conference Series on Public Policy, 50*, 271–324.

Haider, S. J., & Stephens Jr, M. (2007). Is there a retirement-consumption puzzle? Evidence using subjective retirement expectations. *Review of Economics and Statistics, 89*(2), 247–264. https://doi.org/10.1162/rest.89.2.247

Harding, J., Miceli, T. J., & Sirmans, C. F. (2000). Do owners take better care of their housing than renters? *Real Estate Economics, 28*(4), 663–681. https://doi.org/10.1111/1540-6229.00815

Hardy, B., & Ziliak, J. P. (2014). Decomposing trends in income volatility: The "wild ride" at the top and bottom. *Economic Inquiry, 52*(1), 459–476. https://doi.org/10.1111/ecin.12044

Harris, B. H., & Werman, A. (2014). *Retired women at risk for downward social mobility.* Washington, DC: Brookings Institution.

Harvey, C. (2017). *Access to workplace retirement plans by race and ethnicity.* Washington, DC: Fact Sheet. AARP Public Policy Institute.

Haurin, D. R., Parcel, T. L., & Haurin, R. J. (2002). Does homeownership affect child outcomes? *Real Estate Economics, 30*(4), 635–666. https://doi.org/10.1111/1540-6229.t01-2-00053

Haveman, R., Holden, K., Romanov, A., & Wolfe, B. (2007). Assessing the maintenance of savings sufficiency over the first decade of retirement. *International Tax and Public Finance, 14*(4), 481–502.

Herbert, C. E., McCue, D. T., & Sanchez-Moyano, R. (2013). Is homeownership still an effective means of building wealth for low-income and minority households? (Was it ever?). *Homeownership Built to Last, 10*(2), 5–59.

Himmelstein, D. U., Thorne, D., Warren, E., & Woolhandler, S. (2009). Medical bankruptcy in the United States, 2007: Results of a national study. *The American Journal of Medicine, 122*(8), 741–746. https://doi.org/10.1016/j.amjmed.2009.04.012

Himmelstein, D. U., Warren, E., Thorne, D., & Woolhandler, S. (2005). Illness and Injury as Contributors to bankruptcy: Even universal coverage could leave many Americans vulnerable to bankruptcy unless such coverage was more comprehensive than many current policies. *Health Affairs, 24*(Suppl. 1), W5–W63.

Hochguertel, S. (2003). Precautionary motives and portfolio decisions. *Journal of Applied Econometrics, 18*(1), 61–77. https://doi.org/10.1002/jae.658

Holden, S., & Schrass, D. (2016). The role of IRAs in US households' saving for retirement, 2015. *ICI Research Perspective, 22*(1), 1–40.

Huelsman, M. (2015). The debt divide: The racial and class bias behind the "new normal" of student borrowing. *Demos*, pp. 1–34.

Hurd, M., & Rohwedder, S. (2003). *The retirement-consumption puzzle: Anticipated and actual declines in spending at retirement* (No. w9586). Cambridge, MA: National Bureau of Economic Research.

Hurst, E. (2007). *Understanding consumption in retirement: recent developments*. Pension Research Council, The Wharton School. Philadelphia, PA: University of Pennsylvania.

Joint Committee on Taxation & U.S. Congress. (2019). *Background data relating to retirement income*. JCT Report JCX-4-19. Washington, DC: U.S. Congress.

Jud, D., & Winkler, D. (2005). Returns to single-family owner-occupied housing. *Journal of Real Estate Practice and Education, 8*(1), 25–44.

Kalousova, L., & Burgard, S. A. (2013). Debt and foregone medical care. *Journal of Health and Social Behavior, 54*(2), 204–220. https://doi.org/10.1177/0022146513483772

Katz, L. F., & Krueger, A. B. (2017). Documenting decline in US economic mobility. *Science, 356*(6336), 382–383. https://doi.org/10.1126/science.aan3264

Kimball, M. S. (1993). Standard risk aversion. *Econometrica: Journal of the Econometric Society, 61*(3), 589–611. https://doi.org/10.2307/2951719

Kotlikoff, L. J. (1986). *Health expenditures and precautionary savings* (No. w2008). Cambridge, MA: National Bureau of Economic Research.

Krumm, R., & Kelly, A. (1989). Effects of homeownership on household savings. *Journal of Urban Economics, 26*(3), 281–294. https://doi.org/10.1016/0094-1190(89)90002-8

Kurz, C. J., Li, G., & Vine, D. J. (2018). *Are millennials different?* Finance and Economics Discussion Series 2018–080. Washington, DC: Board of Governors of the Federal Reserve System.

Levin, L. (1995). Demand for health insurance and precautionary motives for savings among the elderly. *Journal of Public Economics, 57*(3), 337–367.

Love, D. A., Palumbo, M. G., & Smith, P. A. (2009). The trajectory of wealth in retirement. *Journal of Public Economics, 93*(1–2), 191–208. https://doi.org/10.1016/j.jpubeco.2008.09.003

Lusardi, A., & Mitchell, O. S. (2011). *Financial literacy and planning: Implications for retirement wellbeing* (No. w17078). Cambridge, MA: National Bureau of Economic Research.

Madrian, B. C., & Shea, D. F. (2001). The power of suggestion: Inertia in 401 (k) participation and savings behavior. *The Quarterly Journal of Economics, 116*(4), 1149–1187. https://doi.org/10.1162/003355301753265543

Marshall, S., McGarry, K. M., & Skinner, J. S. (2010). *The risk of out-of-pocket health care expenditure at end of life* (No. w16170). Cambridge, MA: National Bureau of Economic Research.

Minkler, M., & Stone, R. (1985). The feminization of poverty and older women. *The Gerontologist, 25*(4), 351–357. https://doi.org/10.1093/geront/25.4.351

Mitchell, O. S., Mottola, G. R., Utkus, S. P., & Yamaguchi, T. (2006). *The inattentive participant: Portfolio trading behavior in 401 (k) plans.* Michigan Retirement Research Center Research Paper No. WP. (p. 115). Cambridge, MA: National Bureau of Economic Research.

Moore, J. F., & Mitchell, O. S. (2000). Projected retirement wealth and savings adequacy in forecasting retirement needs and retirement wealth. In S. Olivia, P. Mitchell, B. Hammond, & A. M. Rappaport (Eds.), *Forecasting retirement needs and retirement wealth* (pp. 68–94). Philadelphia, PA: Pension Research Council, University of Pennsylvania.

Morduch, J., & Schneider, R. (2017). *The financial diaries: How American families cope in a world of uncertainty.* Princeton, NJ: Princeton University Press.

Munnell, A. H., Hou, W., & Sanzenbacher, G. T. (2018a). National retirement risk index shows modest improvement in 2016. *Center for Retirement Research at Boston College, 18*(1), 1–10.

Munnell, A. H., Hou, W., & Sanzenbacher, G. T. (2018b). *Trends in retirement security by race/ethnicity.* Chestnut Hill, MA: Center for Retirement Research at Boston College.

Munnell, A. H., & Webb, A. (2015). The impact of leakages from 401(k)s and IRAs (IB# 15-2, pp. 1–10). Boston, MA: Center for Retirement Research, Boston College.

Munnell, A. H., Webb, A., & Delorme, L. (2006). *A new national retirement risk index CRR IB No. 48.* Boston, MA: Center for Retirement Research, Boston College.

Mutchler, J., Li, Y., & Xu, P. (2016). *Living below the line: Economic insecurity and older Americans' insecurity, 2016.* Center for Social and Demographic Research on Aging publications No. 13. Boston, MA: University of Massachusetts Boston.

Mutchler, J., Li, Y., & Xu, P. (2017a). *Living below the line: Economic insecurity and older Americans, gender disparities in insecurity, 2016.* Center for Social and Demographic Research on Aging publications No. 19. Boston, MA: University of Massachusetts Boston.

Mutchler, J., Li, Y., & Xu, P. (2017b). *Living below the line: Economic insecurity and older Americans, racial and ethnic disparities in insecurity, 2016.* Boston, MA: University of Massachusetts Boston.

Nakajima, M., & Telyokova, I. (2012). *Home equity in retirement. UCSD working paper.* San Diego, CA: San Diego: University of California.

National Alliance of Caregivers and AARP Public Policy Institute. (2015). *Caregiving in the U.S.* Washington, DC: Author.

Newman, K. S. (2003). *A different shade of grey: Mid-life and beyond in the inner city.* New York, NY: The New Press.

Newman, K. S. (2012). *The accordion family: Boomerang kids, Anxious parents, and the private toll of global competition.* Boston: Beacon Press.

Newman, K. S. (2019). *Downhill from here: Retirement insecurity in the age of inequality.* New York, NY: Metropolitan Books.

Orel, N. A., Ford, R. A., & Brock, C. (2004). Women's financial planning for retirement: The impact of disruptive life events. *Journal of Women & Aging, 16*(3–4), 39–53. https://doi.org/10.1300/J074v16n03_04

Palmer, B. A. (2002). The 2001 GSU/Aon RETIRE project report. *Journal of Financial Service Professionals, 56*(1), 35.

Palumbo, M. G. (1999). Uncertain medical expenses and precautionary saving near the end of the life cycle. *The Review of Economic Studies, 66*(2), 395–421. https://doi.org/10.1111/1467-937X.00092

Pang, G., & Warshawsky, M. (2010). Optimizing the equity-bond-annuity portfolio in retirement: The impact of uncertain health expenses. *Insurance: Mathematics and Economics, 46*(1), 198–209.

Pavalko, E. K., & Artis, J. E. (1997). Women's caregiving and paid work: Causal relationships in late midlife. *The Journals of Gerontology Series B: Psychological Sciences and Social Sciences, 52B*(4), S170–S179. https://doi.org/10.1093/geronb/52B.4.S170

Pew Charitable Trusts. (2017). *Retirement plan access and participation cross generations. A Pew Chart Book.* Washington, DC: Author.

Piketty, T., Saez, E., & Zucman, G. (2017). Distributional national accounts: Methods and estimates for the United States. *The Quarterly Journal of Economics, 133*(2), 553–609. https://doi.org/10.1093/qje/qjx043

Pinquart, M., & Sorensen, S. (2003a). Differences between caregivers and noncaregivers in psychological health and physical health: a meta-analysis. *Psychology of Aging, 8*(2), 250–267. https://doi.org/10.1037/0882-7974.18.2.250

Pinquart, M., & Sorensen, S. (2003b). Associations of stressors and uplifts of caregiving with caregiving with caregiver burden and depressive mood: A meta-analysis. *Journal of Gerontology B: Psychological Science and Social Sciences, 58*(2), 112–P128. https://doi.org/10.1093/geronb/58.2.P112

Pinquart, M., & Sorensen, S. (2006). Gender differences in caregiver stressors, social resources, and health: an updated meta-analysis. *Journal of Gerontology B: Psychological Science and Social Sciences*, 61(1), 33–P45. https://doi.org/10.1093/geronb/61.1.P33

Pinquart, M., & Sorensen, S. (2007). Correlates of physical health of informal caregivers: A meta-analysis. *Journal of Gerontology B: Psychological Science and Social Science*, 62(2), 126–137. https://doi.org/10.1093/geronb/62.2.P126

Porcelli, A. J., & Delgado, M. R. (2009). Acute stress modulates risk taking in financial decision making. *Psychological Science*, 20(3), 278–283.

Poterba, J. M. (2003). Employer stock and 401 (k) plans. *American Economic Review*, 93(2), 398–404. https://doi.org/10.1257/000282803321947416

Poterba, J. M., Venti, S., & Wise, D. (2011). The composition and drawdown of wealth in retirement. *Journal of Economic Perspectives*, 25(4), 95–118. https://doi.org/10.1257/jep.25.4.95

Pratt, J. W., & Zeckhauser, R. J. (1987). Proper risk aversion. *Econometrica: Journal of the Econometric Society*, 55(1), 143–154. https://doi.org/10.2307/1911160

Rainville, C., Skufca, L., & Mehegan, L. (2016). *Family caregiving and out-of-pocket costs: 2016 report. Report for the AARP*. Retrieved fromhttp://www.aarp.org/content/dam/aarp/research/surveys_statistics/ltc/2016/family-caregiving-cost-surveyres-ltc.pdf

Rhee, N. (2013). *The retirement savings crisis*. Washington, DC: National Institute on Retirement Security.

Rhee, N., & Boivie, I. (2015). *The continuing retirement savings crisis*. Washington, DC: National Institute on Retirement Security.

Richard, P., Patel, N., Lu, Y. C., & Alexandre, P. (2018). Self-reported health status and medical debt. *Journal of Financial Counseling and Planning*, 29(1), 36–44. https://doi.org/10.1891/1052-3073.29.1.36

Rohde, N., Tang, K. K., Osberg, L., & Rao, P. (2016). The effect of economic insecurity on mental health: Recent evidence from Australian panel data. *Social Science & Medicine*, 151, 250–258. https://doi.org/10.1016/j.socscimed.2015.12.014

Rohe, W. M., & Lindblad, M. (2013). *Reexamining the social benefits of homeownership after the housing crisis*. Boston: Joint Center for Housing Studies of Harvard University.

Sabelhaus, J., & Henriques, A. M. (2019). *Are disappearing employer pensions contributing to rising wealth inequality?* (No. 2019-02-01). Washington, DC: Board of Governors of the Federal Reserve System.

Scholz, J. K., Seshadri, A., & Khitatrakun, S. (2006). Are Americans saving "optimally" for retirement? *Journal of Political Economy*, 114(4), 607–643. https://doi.org/10.1086/506335

Schwerdt, G. (2005). Why does consumption fall at retirement? Evidence from Germany. *Economics Letters*, 89(3), 300–305. https://doi.org/10.1016/j.econlet.2005.06.014

Scott-Clayton, J., & Li, J. (2016). Black-white disparity in student loan debt more than triples after graduation. *Evidence Speaks Reports, 2*(3), 1–10. Washington, DC: Brookings Institution.

Seifert, R. W., & Rukavina, M. (2006). Bankruptcy is the tip of a medical-debt iceberg: Tracking the number of uninsured Americans is only part of the story: How many insured Americans incur medical debt that deters them from seeking care? *Health Affairs, 25*(Suppl. 1), W89–W92.

Seligman, J. S., & Wenger, J. B. (2006). Asynchronous risk: Retirement savings, equity markets, and unemployment. *Journal of Pension Economics & Finance, 5*(3), 237–255.

Shiller, R. J. (2005). Life-cycle portfolios as government policy. *The Economists' Voice, 2*(1), 1–9.

Shilling, J. D., Sirmans, C. F., & Dombrow, J. F. (1991). Measuring depreciation in single-family rental and owner-occupied housing. *Journal of Housing Economics, 1*(4), 368–383. https://doi.org/10.1016/S1051-1377(05)80018-X

Shin, D., & Solon, G. (2011). Trends in men's earnings volatility: What does the panel study of income dynamics show? *Journal of Public Economics, 95*(7–8), 973–982. https://doi.org/10.1016/j.jpubeco.2011.02.007

Sinai, T., & Souleles, N. S. (2007). *Net worth and housing equity in retirement. NBER working paper No. 13693.* Cambridge, MA: National Bureau of Economic Research.

Sinclair, R. R., & Cheung, J. H. (2016). Money matters: Recommendations for financial stress research in occupational health psychology. *Stress and Health, 32*(3), 181–193. https://doi.org/10.1002/smi.2688

Society of Actuaries. (2018). *Housing in retirement: 2017 risks and process of retirement survey report.* SOA Report. Washington, DC: Society of Actuaries.

Steinbaum, M., & Vaghul, K. (2016). *How the student debt crisis affects African Americans and Latinos. Online report.* Washington, DC: Washington Center for Equitable Growth.

Suari-Andreu, E., Alessie, R., & Angelini, V. (2019). The retirement-savings puzzle reviewed: The role of housing and bequests. *Journal of Economic Surveys, 33*(1), 195–225. https://doi.org/10.1111/joes.12257

Sunden, A. E., & Surette, B. J. (1998). Gender differences in the allocation of assets in retirement savings plans. *The American Economic Review, 88*(2), 207–211.

Thaler, R. H., & Benartzi, S. (2004). Save more tomorrow™: Using behavioral economics to increase employee saving. *Journal of Political Economy, 112*(S1), S164–S187. https://doi.org/10.1086/380085

Turunen, E., & Hiilamo, H. (2014). Health effects of indebtedness: A systematic review. *BMC Public Health, 14*(1), 489. https://doi.org/10.1186/1471-2458-14-489

Van Houtven, C., Coe, B,.N., & Skira, M. (2010). *Effect of informal care on work, wages, and wealth.* Boston College Center for Retirement Research Working Paper. Boston, MA: Center for Retirement Research, Boston College.

VanDerhei, J. (2014). What causes EBRI retirement readiness ratings™ to vary: Results from the 2014 retirement security projection model®. *EBRI Issue Brief*, (396), 1–30.

VanDerhei, J. (2015). Retirement savings shortfalls: Evidence from EBRI's retirement security projection model®. *EBRI Issue Brief*, (410), 1–14.

Venti, S. F., & Wise, D. A. (2004). Aging and housing equity: Another look. In *Perspectives on the economics of aging* (pp. 127–180). Chicago, IL: University of Chicago Press.

Wainer, A., & Zabel, J. (2019). Homeownership and wealth accumulation for low-income households. Article No. 101624. *Journal of Housing Economics*, 47, 1–20.

Walsemann, K. M., & Ailshire, J. A. (2016). Student debt spans generations: Characteristics of parents who borrow to pay for their children's college education. *Journals of Gerontology Series B: Psychological Sciences and Social Sciences*, 72(6), 1084–1089.

Warlick, J. L. (1985). Why is poverty after 65 a woman's problem? *Journal of Gerontology*, 40(6), 751–757. https://doi.org/10.1093/geronj/40.6.751

Warren, T. A., & Warren, T. (2004). *The two-income trap*. New York, NY: Basic Books.

Warshawsky, M. J., & Ameriks, J. (2000). How prepared are Americans for retirement? In O. S. Mitchell, P. Brett Hammond, & A. M. Rappaport (Eds.), *Forecasting retirement needs and retirement wealth* (pp. 33–67). Philadelphia, PA: Pension Research Council, University of Pennsylvania.

Weller, C. E. (2018). *Working-class families are getting hit from all sides. CAP Issue Brief.* Washington, DC: Center for American Progress.

Weller, C. E. (2019, April 22). *People play the generational lottery with their retirement savings accounts.* Forbes.com.

Weller, C. E., & Thompson, J. P. (2018). Wealth inequality more pronounced among Asian Americans than among whites. *Challenge*, *61*(2), 183–202.

Weller, C. E., & Tolson, M. E. (2017). Women's economic risk exposure and savings. *Center for American Progress*, *4*(4), 69–83.

Weller, C. E., & Wenger, J. B. (2009). What happens to defined contribution accounts when labor markets and financial markets move together? *Journal of Aging & Social Policy*, *21*(3), 256–276.

Weller, C., & Wolff, E. (2005). *Retirement income: The crucial role of social security.* Washington, DC: Economic Policy Institute.

Wolff, E. N. (2015). Household wealth inequality, retirement income security, and financial market swings. In C. Weller (Ed.), *Inequality, uncertainty, and opportunity: The varied and growing role of finance in labor relations* (pp. 245–278). Labor and Employment Relations Association Research Volume Series. Ithaca, NY: Cornell University Press.

Wolff, E. N. (2017). *Household wealth trends in the United States, 1962 to 2016: Has middle class wealth recovered?* (No. w24085). Cambridge, MA: National Bureau of Economic Research.

Wolff, J. L., Spillman, B. C., Freedman, V. A., & Kasper, J. D. (2016). A national profile of family and unpaid caregivers who assist older adults with health care activities. *JAMA Internal Medicine*, *176*(3), 372–379.

Yao, R., & Cheng, G. (2017). Millennials' retirement saving behavior: Account ownership and balance. *Family and Consumer Sciences Research Journal*, 46(2), 110–128.

Zeldin, C., & Rukavina, M. (2008). *Borrowing to stay healthy: How credit card debt is related to medical expenses.* New York, NY: Access Project and Demos.

Ziliak, J. P., Hardy, B., & Bollinger, C. (2011). Earnings volatility in America: Evidence from matched CPS. *Labour Economics*, 18(6), 742–754.

CHAPTER 5

With the Wind at Their Backs

Racism and the Amplification of Cumulative Dis/Advantage

Dale Dannefer, Marissa Gilbert, and Chengming Han

ABSTRACT

While interest in the relevance of the cumulative disadvantage perspective has continued to increase steadily over the past several decades, one domain important in the production of inequality has received relatively little attention in analyses of the accumulation of inequality across the life course, and that is the domain of race relations. Focusing on the United States, this chapter explores how federal policies have been designed and implemented to maintain and strengthen the socioeconomic patterning of the American racial hierarchy. It is clear that those who have sought to reinforce existing race-based power relations have had "the wind at their backs" — amplifying political and social interests focused on maintaining the status quo with generic social processes of inequality production. Beginning with Reconstruction and extending across the 20th century and into the present, the convergence of these factors has effectively undermined the prospects for Black workers and families to enjoy opportunities to accumulate resources. White Americans had the opportunity to accumulate wealth, and it has benefited their families for generations, while the opposite effect has happened for Black families who have been systematically excluded from building intergenerational wealth. We discuss several examples of such policies and practices over the past 150 years, including the early plan for "Forty Acres and a Mule," the

Southern Homestead Act, Social Security, the GI Bill, and contemporary predatory student-loan lending. Finally, we end with policy suggestions to address the cumulative disadvantage that Black Americans have been experiencing due to federal U.S. policies.

INTRODUCTION

Since the *Annual Review of Gerontology and Geriatrics* last focused on the age-inequality relation more than 15 years ago (Crystal & Shea, 2002), much has happened in the study of cumulative dis/advantage (CDA). Interest in the topic has continued to grow, evidenced by rigorous theoretical discussions (Crystal, 2006; Dannefer, 2003, 2009, 2018; DiPrete & Eirich, 2006; Pallas & Jennings, 2009; Rigney, 2010), dedicated journal special issues (*Swiss Journal of Sociology, Journals of Gerontology Social Sciences*), and the continued development of an array of related concepts such as weathering (Burton & Whitfield, 2006; Geronimus, 1996; Newman, 2006), the long arm of childhood (Hayward & Gorman, 2004), multiple advantages and disadvantages (Mirowsky & Ross, 2005), and the expansion of the latency-pathways discussion (Kuh & Ben-Schlomo, 2004). Research on CDA has expanded in several directions, including (a) comparative (Aisenbrey & Fasang, 2017; Dannefer & Han, forth; Hoffmann, 2008; Mayer, 2019; Vandecasteele, 2010) and historical (Crystal, Shea, & Reyes, 2016) analyses, (b) increasing evidence that CDA effects follow the socioeconomic (SE) gradient (Ferraro & Shippee, 2009; Mirowsky & Ross, 2003), (c) examining more systematically the role of gender in CDA processes (Giudici & Gauthier, 2013; Widmer & Gauthier, 2013), and (d) considering the relative impact of circumstances encountered at various points in the life course, such as contrasts of childhood and middle adulthood (Dannefer, Kelley-Moore, & Huang, 2016; Hayward & Gorman, 2004). Since 2002, Google Scholar reports more than 17,000 citations to works that link CDA and related concepts to age/life-course topics. The process of scientific discovery that has advanced through these multiple directions of expansion has generated a now-sizeable body of evidence supporting the proposition of increasing inequality over the life course as a pattern that tends to recur across societies and across time, and the field has sought to articulate the multieveled mechanisms through which such empirical patterns are produced at macro-, meso-, and micro-levels of social system dynamics and social interaction.

Despite the scope and multidirectionality of this expansion, one substantive domain with obvious relevance to a full understanding of the social factors and processes regulating CDA has received startlingly little attention, and that is the domain of race relations. Here, as elsewhere, life course theory is lagging far behind research, and with few exceptions, this is true not only for CDA, but for gerontology more generally (Phillipson, 2015, p. 919). Reflecting on the growing attention to the relationship of race, discrimination, and health, Nancy Krieger notes that "Amidst all the debate and new findings, one point stands out: the scientific study of how discrimination harms health requires theoretically grounded methods" (2012, p. 936).

Race relations are especially relevant in understanding CDA in societies such as the United States, where from the beginning race has been deeply and decisively intertwined in the political and economic history as a central axis of inequality, and whose legacy continues to frame conduct and social relations in everyday life. Race has been used extensively in empirical tests of CDA, especially in studies of health disparities, indicating, for example, that racial disparities in functional limitations are associated with differences in socioeconomic status (SES), stressors, and neighborhood conditions (Brown, Hargrove, & Griffith, 2015). Racial health disparities "begin early in life and persist through the life course until advanced ages" (Thorpe, Duru, & Hill, 2015, p. 241). Much research points to the effects of social conditions on racial disparities, such as childhood adversity and poverty, unemployment, and lower education among the Black population (Acevedo-Garcia, Osypuk, McArdle, & Williams, 2008; Kelley-Moore & Huang, 2017; Taylor, 2008). Although this work has been of paramount importance in documenting the power of the SE gradient, it has predominantly used race as an organizing frame for analysis, to allow comparisons between race groups with the general assumption that if the gap between White, Black, and/or Latinx persons grows over time, it likely points to the effect of CDA processes at work. The structural and institutional construction of racial inequality may be acknowledged in these studies but is not fully interrogated.

Our paper will proceed as follows. First, we review relevant aspects of the history of CDA as a guiding perspective for studies of the life course and aging, which reveals some key and unresolved tensions. Second, we explore how the issue of race relations and particularly structural aspects of racism and discrimination in the United States intersects with, and may be used to test, the logic of the CDA perspective and to elaborate its theoretical scope. Third, we illustrate the types of sociohistorical factors that require consideration, if we are to understand how racial discrimination has contributed to patterns of CDA in the United States and that, we suggest, have implications for an understanding of CDA generally.

The Neglect of Race in the Study of CDA

Much of the theoretical literature and most of the empirical analyses documenting the robustness of the phenomenon of CDA have emphasized how it is produced by general social processes and dynamics, such as the stratified reward
structures of K–12 schooling and their reproduction, investments in human capital, organizational dynamics, and so on, with almost no reference to the realities
of structural racism that pervade many of the situations in which these processes
operate in everyday life. Of course these generic dynamics are fundamental to
CDA and are important to explore in their own right, and the literature devoted
to them comprises a foundational and steadily growing body of work. Yet virtually no focused attention has been accorded to the role of race as a structuring
factor in the operation of such processes.

This omission is remarkable for several reasons. First among these is the
simple fact of the centrality of race as a basis of social organization and discrimination, for those who wish to understand the overall dynamics of economic
and health inequality, especially in North America. Second, it is at least equally
remarkable when one considers that the concept of CDA was initially introduced
to the discipline of sociology precisely in a dedicated effort to come to terms
with race inequalities and discrimination in the United States, in Gunnar Myrdal's
landmark work, *An American Dilemma* (1944).

Although Myrdal's work has itself been rightly criticized for its limited analysis of the dynamics surrounding the problem of race (specifically for emphasizing values and cultural dynamics rather than political and economic forces,
and for failing to anticipate the decisive centrality of activism and political struggle in making change [Morris, 2015, pp. 198, 210]), Myrdal must nevertheless
be credited with at least two foundationally important contributions. First, he
clearly recognized the central importance of cumulative processes and CDA in
understanding the problem of race. And second, in dealing with this problem he
introduced what stands as the first explicit and conceptually rigorous treatment
of CDA as a relentless, systemic tendency of social life.

His analysis placed CDA on a sound theoretical foundation that acknowledged the relentless tendency toward amplification—present in all social
interaction processes and social systems—that produces accumulation and
dis-accumulation of resources as inherent to social life. Critiquing basic tenets
of the functionalist or "consensus theory" approach, Myrdal argued that human
social systems tend not to "equilibrate" but to amplify difference, thereby producing inequality in resources and power through ongoing processes of interaction. In so doing, Myrdal made explicit the inherent contradiction between a
paradigmatic approach that recognizes the inherently systemic character of

accumulation on one hand, and the assumptions of the dominant paradigm of sociological functionalism, which view systemic tendencies as tending to stabilize and equilibrate rather than to cumulate and diverge (Dannefer, 2018).

Myrdal thus tied his analysis of CDA and race to a rejection of the placid functionalist approaches that comprised the dominant sociological paradigm when he wrote, and that continue to provide the underlying paradigm for much research in aging and the life course. This is a pathbreaking and enduring contribution that remains valuable, even if Myrdal was himself constrained by some of the other metatheoretical premises and assumptions of the functionalist paradigm.

When one considers the history of discussions of CDA generally, and its relation to race, there are a number of remarkable points to be noted about how Myrdal's pioneering analysis has fared in the sociological discourse on CDA. First, we note that with few exceptions, the entire discourse on CDA (both in general and in relation to age and the life course) has usually been associated not with Myrdal's analysis of race but with Robert Merton's work, and especially his widely cited 1968 paper, "The Matthew Effect in Science." This is all the more striking because Merton's article was published more than 20 years after Myrdal's 1944 publication of *An American Dilemma*. Second, we also note that, while Merton relies heavily on *An American Dilemma* in his classic essay on the self-fulfilling prophecy (1948), he does not credit or cite Myrdal on the matter of cumulative advantage—neither in his initial 1968 "Matthew Effect" paper nor in subsequent work on the topic (1968, 1988). Third is the irony that while Myrdal's initial insights were forged and articulated in a project dedicated to understanding the problem of race, the discourse that has been elaborated around CDA has all but entirely ignored the matter of race relations. By beginning with Merton's 1968 analysis focused on science rather than Myrdal's 1944 analysis focused on race, the CDA literature has managed to avoid a confrontation with the added complexities and challenges introduced when considering the intersection of racial discrimination with structural and political forces.

This neglect of race extends even to the work of those of us who have emphasized the critical social implications of CDA, emphasizing its challenges to the functionalist assumptions that implicitly guide much gerontological research and theorizing (e.g., Crystal, 2006; Dannefer, 1988a, 2003; Pallas & Jennings, 2009). With few exceptions, this work has been conducted with scant attention to Myrdal's formulations (Dannefer, 2018), and with the exception of Daniel Rigney's work (2010, pp. 58–63) with virtually no acknowledgment of the centrality of race in the origins of sociological discussions of the concept of CDA.

CDA can rightly claim to have contributed important dimensions to the life course, drawing attention to sorely neglected theoretical issues of inequality, policy-related issues, social reproduction, and questions bearing on issues of justice, ideology, and practical feasibility. Yet the omission both of Myrdal's pioneering work on emphasizing the relevance of CDA for the problem of race and of race as a central and continuing force in North America must be acknowledged as significant gaps in the current state of this literature. It is clearly a limitation with respect to the general apprehension of societal factors that shape patterns of CDA, but it is more than that. We contend that it also constitutes a limitation in the theoretical development of CDA, specifically with regard to possibilities of change in the face of robust social processes—that is, in the articulation of systemic processes on one hand and the efficacy of deliberate efforts at intervention in social processes on the other.

Systemic Tendencies, Deliberate Interventions, and the Problem of Race

One of the ongoing concerns in discourse on CDA has been the tension between the emphasis on CDA as consisting of "law-like" systemic processes inherent to social systems on one hand, and on the other, the prospects and possibilities for intentional change efforts that might ameliorate or reduce the effect of such systemic tendencies. These two types of forces should not be counterposed as theoretically incompatible; both inevitably operate simultaneously. That is, irrepressible systemic tendencies do not by themselves preclude deliberate interventions to counteract them, any more than gravity precludes space travel. In both cases, deliberate human effort cannot *eradicate* the tendencies that are present in the phenomenon under study, but it can *compensate for* its effects.

Indeed, one primary set of concerns raised by CDA has to do with the practical matter of the *possibilities and prospects for altering* the effects of such systemic tendencies, usually through intentional human interventions designed to reduce adverse effects, such as progressively increasing hardship encountered by those experiencing cycles of cumulative **dis**advantage. Many welfare programs are designed in the service of such objectives, and we generally think of relevant policy interventions as efforts to reduce such adverse effects.

What the history of race relations in the United States offers, by contrast, is another case of the mobilization of intentional human interventions (including interventions in law and policy) to effect change in patterns of CDA, but one with a *precisely opposite intent*: The history of race in the United States is a history of efforts by those in power to protect and strengthen their structural position in society—supercharging their advantage while simultaneously ensuring the continued economic and political exclusion and powerlessness of those already vulnerable. For those concerned to understand more fully the dynamics surrounding CDA, race thus constitutes a case study in considering what can happen when human intentionality is mobilized *to protect and enhance the power of privilege and advantage*, rather than to counter and ameliorate it.

Perhaps especially in the United States, historical and structural aspects of race are clearly integral to the matrix of forces that produce observed outcomes of CDA, as those in power have often engaged in deliberate efforts to protect and nurture White privilege. Yet more than that, this matrix of forces is ignored, and thereby implicitly treated as race-blind and race-neutral in most empirical analyses of CDA presented to date.

Institutionalized Racism, CDA, and Ideology

In what follows, we take some preliminary steps in addressing this neglect by offering a preliminary consideration of the task of integrating the social-structural aspects of the problem of race more centrally into the analysis of the factors underlying CDA. Focusing on the United States, we briefly review instances in which the instruments of law and policy have been deliberately used with the intent of establishing and institutionalizing racist policies and practices, for the purpose of protecting and strengthening White privilege and reinforcing existing structures of inequality. Such deliberate efforts were designed to ensure that race remained integral to the structuring of opportunity, embedding factors that would build race into central social institutions and social dynamics, rules, and practices that would ensure continued stratification, inequality, and race-based exclusion.

These developments obviously have had their origins in intentional human activity designed to enhance the advantage of the powerful by brutal and violent means—beginning with actions of involved in establishing and operating the slave trade, entailing forced trans-Atlantic migration, and an extended period of brutality and enslavement imposed by European colonists. These beginnings created a set of struggles of interest and power that framed subsequent opportunities and life chances, constituting the basis for emergent differences in life-course opportunities in each succeeding generation, that have followed from this neglected yet tragic and formative reality.

In contrast and partly in reaction to this legacy, the official political pronouncements and cultural ideologies framing the public narrative in the United States for more than a half century have been explicitly grounded in a discourse of equal opportunity, advancing a narrative of positive intentions and merit-based ideals that formed the official face of public policy and toward race relations—an emphasis in accordance with a more general legitimation of an ideology of progress (e.g., Bernstein, 1993; Schleshinger, 2002). The foundational realities of the legacy of slavery and the sustained protection of White privilege have been absent from this narrative. While race has remained an undeniable axis of vast inequalities in resources and structured access to resources, the history of the reasons for its importance have received little public or political attention (Katznelson, 2005; Kinder & Kim, 2010; Schwalbe, 2007).

The resultant cultural narrative, emphasizing possibilities of freedom and opportunity and of individual "success" entailed a strong emphasis on putatively universalistic criteria and ideologies of progress and inclusiveness, accompanied by a heavy emphasis on the importance of developing individual characteristics "character," "internal locus of control," "achievement motivation," "resilience," and other putatively desirable traits.

Ideology, Racism, and Sociological Theory

The dominant discourse of twentieth century American sociology fell readily into line with this narrative, with Talcott Parsons vaguely lamenting the continuing challenges of "inclusiveness" (1971) while Ralph Turner characterized the experience of schooling in America as an open "contest"—presented as a refreshingly liberating and meritocratic way to run a school system in contrast to his characterization of traditional "sponsored mobility" schemes. In his depiction of what he perceived as the U.S. educational system's fairness in comparison to more ascriptively based systems (1960, p. 858), Turner describes in detail the contrast between *sponsored* mobility, predicated on a heavy reliance on *ascribed* characteristics and control by elites, often selecting from their own networks, and the centrality of *achieved* status through hard work represented by *contest* mobility. Although this view has been of course widely debunked by scholarship demonstrating the role of schools in reproducing inequality, it remains the official "party line" of public schooling in the United States. This ideology continues to frame the public narrative even as it is tested by obdurate reality of phenomena such as the "school to prison pipeline," which disproportionately targets punitive discipline toward students of color, leading to poorer graduation rates and academic performance records (Hinton, 2017).

The American narratives of opportunity have thus been optimistically keyed to positive expectancies of individual accomplishment and positive mobility. Such emphases have elective affinity not only with the ideology of progress, but also with the idealization of individual conduct of hard work, prudence, and resourcefulness, coupled with unreflected social conformity—thus marginalizing and eclipsing from discussion issues of inequality, unfairness, or exclusionary practices. Such a view renders the ongoing stratifying and caste-reproducing effects of social structure effectively invisible. Yet this has clearly been the case in the study of age and the life course, long dominated by the *functional-developmental nexus* which is described elsewhere as the synergistic bond between the organismic and consensus-based assumptions of the functionalist paradigm in sociology and its uncritical resonance with conventional developmental theory (Dannefer, 1988b, 2000, 2018).

Seen in historical perspective, it is clear that such theorizing has an ideological aspect, as it supports the legitimation of such structures and deflects attention from issues of power differentials and stratification and from the analysis of how social policy supports such interest. Yet even those who have advanced more critical approaches to gerontological analysis, using, for example, political economy and CDA, also appear to be at an early stage of apprehending the scope and impact of the social organization of race.

To illustrate these theoretical points made, we now turn to an examination of some of the ways that race has been rendered nearly invisible in the discourse on CDA processes. We focus specifically on the dramatic differences in inequality among Black and White Americans, which cannot be understood without considering the impact of explicitly designed policies and practices that restricted access to the drivers of economic advancement for Black Americans throughout the 20th century.

Income Inequality and Wealth Inequality

It is increasingly recognized that Black–White income differences, while substantial, fail to capture adequately anything approaching the true magnitude of the legacy of racial discrimination in accounting for the lives of contemporary individuals. One of the ways in which the inadequacy of the examination of income inequality can be seen is by contrasting it with wealth inequality. Compared to income, wealth is a more telling characteristic with which to appraise inequality for several reasons. It may afford access to social and cultural capital that has been linked to intergenerational transmission, and, of course, wealth holds the power to generate more wealth (Darity et al., 2018). Wealth inequality is more stable and enduring than income as a general characteristic. Scholars prefer wealth inequality than income inequality because household wealth is more comprehensive, not only does wealth included accumulative possessions in the past, it also indicates the inheritance from older generation (Banks, Blundell, & Smith, 2004; Gittleman & Wolff, 2004; Hamilton & Kohli, 2003, 2004, 2005; Shapiro, 2004).

Such factors add importance to the even more basic fact that wealth inequality is vastly greater than income inequality. Based on results of a Pew Report survey, Shapiro, Meshede, and Osoro report that in 2009, "the median wealth of White families was $113,149 compared with $6,325 for Latino families and $5,677 for Black families" (2013, p. 1, see also Kochhar, Fry, & Taylor, 2011). In other words, Black family wealth is almost exactly 5% of White wealth. Moreover, these researchers report that this dramatic difference was aggravated by the Great

Recession of 2007–2009. By contrast, income for Black men is about 70% that for White males. Although this is a large and glaring difference, it is modest in comparison to the wealth difference. Wealth is, of course, not just a stand-alone indicator; it is bound up with other matters such as access to higher education and opportunities for home ownership and entrepreneurship—all of which should be relevant to the issue of equal opportunity, according to general assertions of broadly shared cultural values and in some cases, official policy pronouncements. Even middle class Black families who earn competitive salaries frequently have much less wealth and disposable income, as they continue to pay the cost of a lack of intergenerational wealth (Darity et al., 2018; Shapiro, 2004, 2017).

Of course, attention to inequalities in wealth and privilege may have been obscured and deflected by the same forces that appeal to those who wish to minimize the significance of inequality generally, as discussed earlier. Thus, it is perhaps not entirely surprising that the subject of inheritance and the enormous differences in familial wealth available to youth of different backgrounds has received little attention in public discourse, nor has it appeared in many strands of influential academic theorizing.

Since wealth is generally based on family units, it has clear implications for the resources available to offspring at the beginning of the life course. The vast differences in assets reported earlier make plain the disadvantage in SE life chances of Black as compared with White youth in the United States.

It is important to consider these realities in view of the dominant narrative of the "American Dream"—a narrative of open horizons of opportunity and merit-based rewarding of individual efforts and accomplishment, in which social structure is rendered invisible. It is also important to contemplate them when research invites interpretations of these differences in individualistic terms (i.e., based on individual prudence and responsibility, or other aspects of "character", or even genes [see, e.g., Caspi, Moffitt, Newman, & Silva, 1996; see also Dannefer, 1999). Such an interpretation is the default setting when race is introduced into the study of age and life course simply as an individual characteristic.

This narrative of individual possibility, responsibility, and potential accomplishment ignores and obscures the harsh and overdetermined realities of deliberate and sustained practices of racial discrimination embodied in social policies. In other words, although structural racism was "baked in" to U.S. policies that were designed to promote economic expansion and social mobility throughout the 20th century, these origins were quickly forgotten and replaced with meritocratic and individual effort explanations for SE success. This nearly fully assured a White upperclass and a perpetual Black underclass, all framed as either accomplishment or failure in a "race blind" economic system. We outline some of these policies in the next section.

Social Policy and the Protection of White Privilege

While a full exposition of the history of legal and economic arrangements that are responsible for current race-based inequalities is beyond the scope of this paper, we offer a first step toward such an appraisal by reviewing examples from three different time periods, demonstrating the resilience of laws, policies, and practices which have helped ensure the continued exclusion of Black Americans from mainstream structures of opportunities since the official abolition of slavery. In some cases, these efforts were intentional, and they have been highly successful in realizing their intended effects: (a) the initial postslavery promises and hopes represented by the ideal captured in the famous slogan, "forty acres and a mule," and the Southern Homestead Act, (b) in the mid-20th century the establishment of Social Security; and the post-World War II GI Bill, and in the 21st century, the disproportionate impact on Black students and graduates of the student loan crisis.

"Forty Acres and a Mule" and the Southern Homestead Act

The promise of immediate reconciliation for the intentional deprivation of resources and humanity to Black Americans after the time of enslavement was dim but did in fact exist. After slavery was abolished, perhaps half a million or more acres of land from previous plantations were collected by the Freedman's Bureau with the assistance of a Union general, William T. Sherman (Darity, 2008). The general also encouraged the army to offer their mules to the freed Blacks to use on their new land (Myers, 2005). The Freedman's Bureau and Sherman began working together to discuss donating the confiscated land, located along the coast of several southern states, to former slaves (Conley, 2002). As formerly enslaved Blacks had few, if any, opportunities to own land of their own, this promise inspired great hope because it envisioned a new era of economic empowerment for Blacks in the South.

These efforts proved to be short-lived, and effectively stillborn. As U.S. President Andrew Johnson opposed this initiative and, at least partly through his influence, the land that had been promised to freed slaves was instead offered to White northerners and previous slave owners in the south who then outsourced the labor on the farms to Black workers, who were severely undercompensated leading to the institutionalization of share cropping (Conley, 2002). In a second effort to provide opportunities for farm ownership to freed slaves Congress passed the Southern Homestead Act of 1866, which followed shortly after the failed promise of forty acres and a mule (Darity, 2008). The Act offered farmland that was not already privately owned, and in turn had no potential of successful harvest seasons due to subpar soil quality (Gates, 1940). The Black/White wealth disparity has long been ingrained into the history of the United

States and unrealized promises from the U.S. government after the abolition of slavery represent early instances in the now-familiar succession of policies that squelched opportunities and hopes for prosperity and the opportunity to accumulate resources by Black Americans.

Henry Louis Gates, Jr. demonstrated the cumulative advantage of having received property and economic freedom immediately following the Civil War in his unique effort to trace families of current successful Black Americans such as astronaut Mae Jemison and celebrity Oprah Winfrey. The vast majority of these Black Americans who were or are at the top of their professional fields came from families who were able to obtain property very early in the 20th century (https://www.nytimes.com/2007/11/18/opinion/18gates.html). While these cases are clearly the exception and not the rule for Black Americans, it is a clear indication of the importance of access to vehicles of wealth and its intergenerational accumulative effects.

Social Security and the GI Bill

Second, consider two notable mid-century uses of policy to provide economic support to citizens. First, Social Security, launched in 1935, stands as one of the longest running social welfare projects of modern history (Katznelson, 2005) and is, of course, still widely popular. It has provided benefits to scores of millions of Black older adults as well as White older adults, accomplishing one of the original goals of Social Security: to protect older adults and those unable to work in the United States. Yet access to its benefits has not been race-neutral and from its very beginning was framed by and shadowed with race-related politics.

These circumstances resulted from several interrelated factors at play in the original establishment of Social Security, driven by political expediency and the obdurate ideology of racism. Although Social Security seemingly gave everyone equal opportunity to accumulate wages, the policy carefully and deliberately excluded certain lines of work that were commonly divided along racial groups. The program intentionally disqualified agricultural and domestic laborers, two fields of employment that were most commonly available for Black Americans to find work (Katznelson, 2005; Poole, 2006) while navigating the racial politics of the labor market in the deep South. Although Southern Democrats in Congress represented aging and increasingly poor populations in desperate need of relief, these "Dixiecrat" legislators were even more concerned to ensure the preservation of the contours of the Antebellum arrangements and social order that supported White privilege. To win their votes, a compromise was struck that excluded from eligibility types of work typically performed by Blacks (i.e., agricultural and domestic labor), allowing southern and some northern Democrats to maintain their interests in White supremacy while seemingly still supporting the older community they deemed worthy of assistance. Moreover, since individual state governments held the power to decide how the policy was carried out, much of the intended benefit never reached Black citizens (Katznelson, 2005, pp. 44–45).

The Social Security Act also was also designed to provide relief to temporarily unemployed workers. However, this benefit was similarly riddled with racial undertones. Many Black workers were excluded from eligibility, as Social Security's program benefited only to workers of large companies or industries (Poole, 2006, p. 69). The millions of Black Americans receiving limited Social Security benefits, combined with the silent portion working in domestic and agricultural labor and hence excluded from eligibility, continued to widen the accumulation of wealth disparity racially embedded restrictions.

It is true that, despite these deliberate exclusionary practices, more Black employees were assisted through this program than through any previous policy. At the same time, however, the benefits they received were substantially less than that of their White counterparts, further depriving them of opportunities to accumulate more wealth (Katznelson, 2005; Poole, 2006).

While not characterized by the deliberate exclusionary efforts that characterized the Social Security law, the GI Bill offers a contemporaneous example of embedded race discrimination in state-sanctioned governmental policies. This GI Bill (Servicemen's Readjustment Act of New Deal) provided avenues for veterans to gain access to housing, college educations, and the overall American Dream, and has been generally deemed to be widely successful. Specifically, veterans securing housing heavily contributed to the economic success of the growing middle class. It is perhaps noteworthy that the lone exception to the generally robust pattern of increasing family income inequality with increasing age has been attributed to the GI Bill (Dannefer & Han, forthcoming; Falletta & Dannefer, 2014).

While both White and Black veterans were entitled to benefits from these policies, the reality in practice often gave a clear advantage to White veterans (Katznelson, 2005, pp. 121–122). As with Social Security, some aspects of the program were administered at the state level, a practice which ". . . ensured discriminatory treatment for Blacks" (Katznelson, 2005, p. 128). Institutionalized racist policies such as redlining, denying Black veterans access to mortgage loans, and the racial politics of White higher education institutions marginalized Black veterans.

Federal and state policies over the past decades in the United States have maintained that they are neutrally providing equal access for all. Although neither Social Security nor the GI Bill explicitly mentions the discriminatory practices toward Black Americans, these policies are covertly rooted in what Bonilla-Silva

(2006, pp. 1–2) has identified as "colorblind racism"—based on the assumption that the problem of racism has now been solved, and that equal opportunity as a societal goal has been essentially realized and those who do not succeed do so because of their own doings or their own lack of effort.

Contemporary Forms of Racial Discrimination and Exclusion: The Case of Student Loan Debt and Wealth

Institutional "color blind" racism is still prevalent today, manifested in multiple domains, including the school to prison pipeline, the disproportionately adverse costs borne by Black victims of predatory lending in the 2008 mortgage crisis, and in the ongoing student loan crisis.

As more Black Americans pursue college degrees, many—like White students—find it necessary to take out student loans. However, because of the lack of personal and familial resources, Black students take more student loans out than their White counterparts. According to the data from the National Center for Education Statistics (NCES), nearly 86.8% of Black students need federal student loans to enroll in a 4-year public college, while the percentage for White student is 59.9% (Safier, 2018). Although it may not be surprising that Black graduates leave college with more debt, a recent analysts indicates that the race disparity is dramatic, and much greater than many analyses expected: Scott-Clayton and Li (2016) found that the accumulation of debt by Black graduates (bachelor's degree) in a 1997 cohort was nearly triple that of White graduates.

Moreover, Black graduates receive less return in the labor market for their postsecondary degree than do White graduates (Gaddis, 2015). Essentially Black students enter higher education institutions with less wealth, leading to more student loan debt, only to graduate and take longer paying back this debt. The cyclical effects of small amounts of wealth accumulation and intergenerational wealth exchange, continue to contribute to the accumulation of disadvantages for Blacks in modern times.

Numerous scholars have argued that these general difficulties have been exacerbated by the predatory and aggressive targeting of students of color by for-profit universities. The early claims that for-profit colleges would act as a supplement and sometimes lower-cost alternative to the public education (Chung, 2012) that could expand educational and labor market opportunities, have not been realized. Indeed, degrees from for-profit colleges have proven to be less rewarding—often dramatically so—than a nonprofit college degree (Lynch, Engle, & Cruz, 2010) and such institutions have been accused of defrauding students (Bonadies, Rovenger, Connor, Shum, & Merrill, 2018). To the extent that such accusations have merit, they may especially apply to the effects of such institutions for students of color.

Because of the often inflated tuition rates, the cost of for-profit schools compel many students to apply for student loans (Mullin, 2010). Large student loan debts are daunting for everyone, but especially so for Black graduates who face higher rates of unemployment (Jones & Schmitt, 2014) and earn less than White peer graduates (Zhang, 2008). In their analysis of the targeting of Black and Brown communities by for-profit schools, Seamster and Charron-Chénier (2017) argue that encouraging high rates of student loan debts is an act of "predatory inclusion" in which access to a "resource" (i.e., a student loan) is granted from institutional powers (in this case universities) to a group of marginalized people who have been systemically and historically excluded from this resource. Thus the gain from the access to the resources, the financial benefits of a college degree, is almost completely eliminated.

Cumulating White Advantage

By ensuring the continued substantial and institutionalized stratification of opportunities by race, one legacy of policies and arrangements such as those discussed previously has arguably been the strengthening of the "White racial frame" that has been integral to the historical development of cultural dynamics of the United States (Feagin, 2013). This frame asserts the invisible normalcy associated with Whiteness provides a continued privilege for White Americans while simultaneously disadvantaging non-White Americans. This privilege is noticeable in the aforementioned government policy and continues into contemporary social processes. From employment discrimination (Pager & Shepherd, 2008) to residential segregation (Massey & Denton, 1993), Black Americans have been continuously marginalized and excluded from upward mobility while the privilege associated with white skin continues to reproduce covert racially driven inequality.

Challenging Cumulative White Advantage: Policy Proposals

We have seen clearly in the foregoing how effectively deliberate human action can be used, and has often been used intentionally, to realize the goals of those who have sought to protect White privilege and use law and policies as instruments to safeguard traditional patterns of segregation and exclusion, policies that have reinforced the systemic tendencies for inequality to increase among age peers over their collective life course, and sharpened their differentiation along the lines of race. This convergence of systematic tendencies and existing power arrangements has meant, not surprisingly, that those so positioned have found that the wind is at their back. In this context, what possibilities exist for countering, instead of reinforcing, those same systemic tendencies? A wide range of responses has been proposed and considered over recent decades, of course, and not all are equally promising. In the brief space remaining, we suggest two recently proposed responses that warrant consideration, when those concerned with the relentless tendencies of CDA contemplate strategies of amelioration—(a) some form of *reparations* and (b) the investment in *baby bonds*. These are not new ideas, of course, but such notions have been conspicuously absent from discussions of CDA.

First, as a response to the discriminatory formulas embedded in policies and practices just reviewed and the associated wealth gap, a program of *reparations* could be implemented. Reparations can be carried out in many forms, one of which being direct financial compensation to Black Americans for their unpaid work and the role the federal and state government have played in their exploitation and exclusion from social welfare benefits. Because of the United States' individualistic ideology interwoven with colorblind racism, reparations, though sensibly a solution after examining the unjust distribution of power, wealth, and social boundaries, are unlikely to be fully supported by the majority of society.

A second policy proposal, offered by economists Darrick Hamilton and William Darity, Jr. (2010), is the notion of "baby bonds." Advocates for baby bonds argue that they could efficiently result in greater racial equity while appeasing to the colorblind racism embedded in policy change. A baby bond, as argued by Hamilton and Darity, averaging $20,000 and growing upward toward $60,000 in severe wealth-deprived families, could generate wealth in upcoming generations directly, with an investment in capital at birth. As proposed, baby bonds would be introduced as a benefit for all children whose family's wealth is below the national median of wealth accumulated by families in the United States. However, with the disproportionate experience of wealth deprivation endured by Black families, this policy could effectively address racial equity.

CONCLUSION

A challenge that cumulative dis/advantage and gerontological scholars must confront moving forward is pushing beyond race as an individual characteristic in the life course discussion, and recognizing it instead as an explanatory force rooted in the structure of institutions and social organization. Much attention has been devoted to the salutary impact of pension and retirement programs exemplified by Social Security, which has dramatically reduced old-age poverty and perhaps inequality over the past 75 years. Yet in gerontology, very little attention has been devoted to the ways in which the Social Security Act itself has served to reproduce and sustain patterns of racial discrimination and exclusion, contributing to the maintenance of patterns of inequality, and strengthening cumulative dis/advantage, nor to how such programmatic innovations earlier in the life course could mitigate old-age inequality and its health consequences.

Navigating through the world as a Black American is thus, inevitably, a matter of navigating a legacy of oppression and economic exclusion. Though the forms this takes may differ across cohorts, the enduring structure of racialized disadvantage remains an obdurate constant. By contrast, being a White American carries inherent privilege, and law and social policies have long been utilized as deliberate instruments to protect and enhance that privilege.

We have seen, then, that human intentionality directed toward producing particular outcomes can indeed alter effects of the inherent, systemic tendencies toward the generation of CDA that are present in any social system play out in people's lives. To be more specific, in the case of race relations, we have seen that intentionality can alter such systemic tendencies not by resisting or counteracting them, but by deliberately reinforcing them. We have seen that the deliberate, agentic efforts of the powerful and privileged to exclude Black citizens from opportunities were successful in achieving their goals in ways that clearly amplified or supercharged inherent tendencies toward CDA.

We have also seen that governmental efforts to reduce systemic tendencies by providing a near-universal social safety net in the form of Social Security have for Blacks been a two-edged sword. Simultaneously, Social Security both (a) broad-based benefits for the population generally including Black Americans and (b) contained within its founding rules and patterns of implementation mechanisms by which the overall structure of race-based inequality could be preserved.

Indeed, when one considers the overall development of historical events and their context, it is impressive to consider how effectively the social history of the United States reflects the intentions of embodied in programs implemented by those in power, who often sought deliberately to nourish and reproduce White privilege. It is of crucial importance to remember and understand this legacy, for those interested in using law and policy as instruments to address the effects of CDA, and life course scholars more generally.

ACKNOWLEDGMENTS

We thank Stephen Crystal, Angela O'Rand, and Chris Phillipson and the editors of ARGG for helpful comments on an earlier draft of this paper.

REFERENCES

Acevedo-Garcia, D., Osypuk, T. L., McArdle, N., & Williams, D. R. (2008). Toward a policy-relevant analysis of geographic and racial/ethnic disparities in child health. *Health Affairs, 27*(2). published online

Aisenbrey, S., & Fasang, A. (2017). The interplay of work and family trajectories over the life course: Germany and the United States in comparison. *American Journal of Sociology, 122*(5), 1448–1484.

Banks, J., Blundell, R., & Smith, J. P. (2004). Wealth portfolios in the United Kingdom and the United States. In D. Wise (Ed.), *Perspectives on the economics of aging* (pp. 205–246). Chicago, IL: University of Chicago Press.

Baum, S., & Payea, K. (2011, November). *Education: Enrollment, prices, student aid and outcomes.* Retrieved from www.collegeboard.org/trends

Bernstein, I. (1993). *Promises kept: John F. Kennedey's new frontier.* New York, NY: Oxford.

Bonadies, G., Rovenger, J., Connor, E., Shum, B., & Merrill, T. (2018, July 30). *For-profit schools' predatory practices and students of color: A mission to enroll rather than educate. Harvard law review blog administrative law, Civil rights, Education law.* Retrieved from https://blog.harvardlawreview.org/for-profit-schools-predatory-practices-and-students-of-color-a-mission-to-enroll-rather-than-educate/

Bonilla-Silva, E. (2006). *Racism without racists: Color-blind racism and the persistence of racial inequality in the United States.* New York, NY: Rowman & Littlefield Publishers.

Brown, T. H., Hargrove, T. W., & Griffith, D. M. (2015). Racial/Ethnic disparities in men's health: Examining psychosocial mechanisms. *Family Community Health, 38*(4), 307–318. https://doi.org/10.1097/FCH.0000000000000080

Burton, L., & Whitfield, K. (2006). Health, aging and America's poor: Ethnographic insights on family co-morbidity and cumulative disadvantage. In J. Baars, D. Dannefer, C. Phillipson, & A. Walker (Eds.), *Aging, globalization and inequality* (pp. 215–230). Amityville, NY: Baywood.

Caspi, A., Moffitt, T. E., Newman, D. L., & Silva, P. A. (1996). Behavioral observations at age 3 years predict adult psychiatric disorders: Longitudinal evidence from a birth cohort. *Archives of General Psychiatry, 53*, 1033–1039.

Chung, A. S. (2012). Choice of for-profit college. *Economics of Education Review, 31*(6), 1084–1101.

Conley, D. (2002). Forty acres and a mule: What if America pays reparations? *Contexts, 1*(3), 13–20.

Crystal, S. (2006). Dynamics of late-life inequality: Modeling the interplay of health disparities, economic resources, and public policies. In J. Baars, D. Dannefer, C. Phillipson, & A. Walker (Eds.), *Aging, globalization and inequality: The new critical gerontology* (pp. 205–213). New York: Baywood Publishing Company.

Crystal, S., & Shea, D. (Eds.). (2002). *Annual review of gerontology and geriatrics.* New York, NY: Springer Publishing Company.

Crystal, S., Shea, D., & Reyes, A. (2016). Cumulative advantage, cumulative disadvantage, and evolving patterns of late-life inequality. *The Gerontologist, 57*(5), 910–920. https://doi.org/10.1093/geront/gnw056

Dannefer, D. (1988a). Differential gerontology and the stratified life course: Conceptual and methodological issues. M. P. Lawton & G. Maddox (Eds.), *Annual review of gerontology & geriatrics* (Vol, 8, pp. 3–36). New York, NY: Springer Publishing Company.

Dannefer, D. (1988b). What's in a name?: An account of the neglect of variability in the study of aging. In J. E. Birren & V. L. Bengtson (Eds.), *Emergent theories of aging* (pp. 356–384). New York, NY: Springer Publishing Company.

Dannefer, D. (1999). Neoteny, Naturalization and other constituents of human development. In C. D. Ryff & V. W. Marshall (Eds.), *The self and society of aging processes* (pp. 67–93). New York, NY: Springer Publishing Company.

Dannefer, D. (2000). Paradox of opportunity: Education, work, and age integration in the United States and Germany. *The Gerontologist, 40*(3), 282–286.

Dannefer, D. (2003). Cumulative advantage/disadvantage and the life course: Cross-fertilizing age and social science theory. *Journals of Gerontology Social Sciences, 58B,* S327–S337.

Dannefer, D. (2009). Stability, homogeneity, agency: Cumulative dis-advantage and problems of theory. *Swiss Journal of Sociology, 35*(2), 193–210.

Dannefer, D. (2018). Systemic and reflexive: Foundations of cumulative dis/advantage and life-course processes. *The Journals of Gerontology: Series B, 118, 1*–15. https://doi.org/10.1093/geronb/gby118

Dannefer, D., & Han, C. (forthcoming). Process, policy and life course patterning: Life course patterning. In *Current debates in aging and the life course; Policy.* Routledge.

Dannefer, D., Han, C., & Yu, J. (forthcoming). Inequality across time: Social change, biography and the life course. In *Routledge international handbook of inequalities and the life course.*

Dannefer, D., Kelley-Moore, J., & Huang, W. (2016). Opening the social: Sociological imagination in life course studies. In M. J. Shanahan, J. T. Mortimer, & M. K. Johnson (Eds.), *Handbook of the life course voume II* (pp. 87–110). Cham, Switzerland: Springer International Publishing. https://doi.org/10.1007/978-3-319-20880-0_4

Darity, W., Jr. (2008). Forty acres and a mule in the 21st century. *Social Science Quarterly, 89*(3), 656–664.

Darity, W., Jr., Hamilton, D., Paul, M., Aja, A., Price, A., Moore, A., & Chiopris, C. (2018, April). *What we get wrong about closing the racial wealth gap. Samuel duBois cook center on social equity and insight center for community economic development.* Retrieved from https://socialequity.duke.edu/portfolio-item/what-we-get-wrong-about-closing-the-racial-wealth-gap/

DiPrete, T. A., & Eirich, G. M. (2006). Cumulative advantage as a mechanism for inequality: A review of theoretical and empirical developments. *Annual Review of Sociology, 32,* 271–297. https://doi.org/10.1146/annurev.soc.32.061604.123127

Falletta, L., & Dannefer, D. (2014). The life course and the social organization of age. In J. Macleod, E. J. Lawler, & M. Schwalbe (Eds.), *Handbook of the social psychology of inequality* (pp. 607–625). New York, NY: Springer.

Feagin, J. R. (2013). *The white racial frame: Centuries of racial framing and counter-framing.* New York, NY: Routledge.

Ferraro, K. F., & Shippee, T. P. (2009). Aging and cumulative inequality: How does inequality get under the skin? *The Gerontologist, 49*(3), 333–343. https://doi.org/10.1093/geront/gnp034

Gaddis, S. M. (2015). Discrimination in the credential society: An audit study of race and college selectivity in the labor market. *Social Forces, 93*(4), 1451–1479.

Gates, P. W. (1940). Federal land policy in the south 1866-1888. *The Journal of Southern History, 6*(3), 303–330.

Geronimus, A. T. (1996). Black/white differences in the relationship of maternal age to birthweight: A population-based test of the weathering hypothesis. *Social Science & Medicine, 42*(4), 589–597.

Gittleman, M., & Wolff, E. (2004). Racial differences in patterns of wealth accumulation. *Journal of Human Resources, 39*(1), 193–227.

Giudici, F., & Gauthier, J. (2013). Occupational trajectories after childbirth 50. *Ausdruck, 14*(2), 95–116.

Hamilton, D., & Darity, W., Jr. (2010). Can "Baby Bonds" eliminate the racial wealth gap in putative post-racial America? *Review of Black Political Economy, 37*(3–4), 207–216.

Hayward, M. D., & Gorman, B. K. (2004). The long arm of childhood: The influence of early-life social conditions on men's mortality. *Demography, 41*, 87–107.

Hinton, E. (2017). *From the war on poverty to the war on crime: The making of mass incarceration in America.* Boston MA: Harvard University Press.

Hoffmann, R. (2008). *Socioeconomic differences in old age mortality.* New York, NY: Springer.

Jones, J., & Schmitt, J. (2014, May). *A college degree is no guarantee.* Washington, DC: Center for Economic and Policy Research. Retrieved from cepr.net/publications/reports/a-college-degree-is-no-guarantee

Katznelson, I. (2005). *When affirmative action was white: An untold history of racial inequality in twentieth-century America.* New York, NY: WW Norton & Company.

Kelley-Moore, J., & Huang, W. (2017). The "Good Times" cohort in later-life: Black–white differences in pathways to functional limitations. *Research on Aging, 39*(4), 526–548.

Kinder, D. R., & Kim, C. D. (2010). *Us against them: Ethnocentric foundations of american opinion.* Chicago, IL: The University of Chicago Press.

Kochhar, R., Fry, R., & Taylor, P. (2011). *Wealth gaps rise to record highs between whites, blacks, and hispanics.* Washington, DC: Pew Social & Demographic Trends.

Kohli, M. (2003). *Intergenerational family transfers in aging societies.* Condensed version in American Sociological Association, Section on Aging and the Life Course, Newsletter, Fall 2003 (pp. 4–5).

Kohli, M. (2004). Intergenerational transfers and inheritance: A comparative view. In M. Silverstein (Ed.), *Annual review of gerontology and geriatrics Vol 24 – intergenerational relations across time and place* (pp. 266–289). New York, NY: Springer Publishing Company.

Kohli, M. (2005). Generational changes and generational equity. In M. L. Johnson, V. L. Bengtson, P. G.Coleman, & T. B. L. Kirkwood (Eds.), *The Cambridge handbook of age and aging* (pp. 518–526). Cambridge, NY: Cambridge University Press.

Krieger, N. (2012). Methods for the scientific study of discrimination and health: An ecosocial approach. *American Journal of Public Health, 102*(5), 936–944. https://doi.org/10.2105/AJPH.2011.300544

Kuh, D., & Ben-Schlomo, Y. (2004). *A life-course approach to chronic disease epidemiology.* Oxford: Oxford University Press.

Lynch, M., Engle, J., & Cruz, A. (2010, November). *Subprime opportunity: The unfulfilled promise of for-profit colleges and universities.* Washington, DC: Education Trust. Retrieved from http://www.edtrust.org/sites/edtrust.org/files/publications/files/Subprime_report.pdf

Massey, D. S., & Denton, N. A. (1993). *American apartheid: Segregation and the making of the underclass.* Cambridge, MA: Harvard University Press.

Mayer, K. U. (2019, September). *Life courses and social inequality: Comparative perspectives.* Paper presented at the Society of Longitudinal and life-course studies. Berlin-Brandenburg, Germany.

Merton, R. K. (1948). The self-fulfilling prophecy. *The Antioch Review, 8*(2), 193–210.

Merton, R. K. (1968). The Matthew effect in science: The reward and communication system of science. *Science, 199,* 55–63.

Merton, R. K. (1988). The Matthew effect in science, II: Cumulative advantage and the symbolism of intellectual property. *ISIS, 79*(4), 606–623.

Mirowsky, J., & Ross, E. (2003). *Education, social status, and health.* New York, NY: Aldine de Gruyte.

Mirowsky, J., & Ross, E. (2005). Education, age, and the cumulative advantage in health. *Ageing International, 30*(1), 27–62. https://doi.org/10.1007/BF02681006

Morris, A. (2015). *The scholar denied: W.E.B. duBois and the birth of modern sociology.* Berkeley: University of California Press.

Mullin, C. M. (2010). *Just how similar? Community colleges and the for-profit sector.* AACC Policy Brief 2010-04PBL. American Association of Community Colleges (NJ1). Retrieved from https://files.eric.ed.gov/fulltext/ED522994.pdf

Myers, B. (2005). *Sherman's field order No. 15. New georgia encyclopedia.* Retrieved from https://www.georgiaencyclopedia.org/articles/history-archaeology/shermans-field-order-no-15 on 2017, June 08

Myrdal, G. (1944). *An American dilemma: The negro problem and modern democracy.* New York, NY; London: Harper and Brothers.

Newman, K. S. (2006). *A different shade of gray: Midlife and beyond in the inner city.* New York, NY: New Press.

Pager, D., & Shepherd, H. (2008). The sociology of discrimination: Racial discrimination in employment, housing, credit, and consumer markets. *Annual Review of Sociology, 34,* 181–209.

Pallas, A. M., & Jennings, J. L. (2009). Cumulative knowledge about cumulative advantage. *Swiss Journal of Sociology, 35,* 211–229.

Parsons, T. (1971). *The system of modern societies.* Englewood Cliffs, NJ: Prentice-Hall.

Phillipson, C. (2015). Placing ethnicity at the center of studies of later life: Theoretical perspectives and empirical challenges. *Ageing & Society, 35*(5), 917–934.

Poole, M. (2006). *The segregated origins of social security: African Americans and the welfare state*. Chapel Hill, NC: University of North Carolina Press.

Rigney, D. (2010). *The Matthew effect: How advantage begets further advantage*. New York, NY: Columbia University Press.

Safier, R. (2018, September 17). *Study: Student loans weigh the heaviest on black and hispanic students*. Retrieved from https://studentloanhero.com/featured/study-student-loans -weigh-heaviest-black-hispanic/

Schleshinger, A. M. (2002). *One thousand days: John F. Kennedy in the white house*. New York, NY: Mariner Books.

Schwalbe, M. (2007). *Rigging the game: How inequality is reproduced in everyday life*. New York, NY: Oxford University Press.

Scott-Clayton, J., & Li, J. (2016). Black-white disparity in student loan debt more than triples after graduation. *Economic Studies*, 2(3), 1–9. Retrieved from https://vtechw orks.lib.vt.edu/handle/10919/83265

Seamster, L., & Charron-Chénier, R. (2017). Predatory inclusion and education debt: Rethinking the racial wealth gap. *Social Currents*, 4(3), 199–207.

Shapiro, T. M. (2004). *The hidden cost of being African American: How wealth perpetuates inequality*. New York, NY: Oxford University Press.

Shapiro, T. M. (2017). *Toxic inequality: How America's wealth gap destroys mobility, deepens the racial divide, and threatens our future*. New York, NY: Basic Books.

Taylor, M. G. (2008). Timing, accumulation, and the black/white disability gap in later life: A test of weathering. *Research on Aging*, 30(2), 226–250.

Thorpe, R. J., Duru, O. K., & Hill, C. V. (2015). Advancing racial/ethnic minority men's health using a life course approach. *Ethnicity & Disease*, 25(3), 241–244.

Turner, R. (1960). Sponsored and contest mobility and the school system. *American Sociological Review*, 25, 855–867.

Vandecasteele, L. (2010). Life course risks or cumulative disadvantage? the structuring effect of social stratification determinants and life course events on poverty transitions in europe. *European Sociological Review*, 27(2), 246–263.

Widmer, E. D., & Gauthier, J. A. (2013). Cohabitational trajectories. In R. Levy & E. D. Widmer (Eds.), *Gendered life courses* (pp. 53–70). Berlin: Lit Verlag.

Zhang, L. (2008). Gender and racial gaps in earnings among recent college graduates. *The Review of Higher Education*, 32(1), 51–72.

CHAPTER 6

Social Rights of the Elderly as Part of the New Human Rights Agenda

Noncontributory Pensions and Civil Society in Mexico

Ronald J. Angel and Verónica Montes de Oca

ABSTRACT

Today, social rights, which include the basic material requirements for a dignified life, are at the core of the new human rights agenda. Recent international conventions that address the problems of poverty, discrimination, isolation, and social exclusion among older persons have produced general principles that affirm their social, as well as political rights. Retirement security and healthcare represent two of the core pillars of the welfare state as it evolved during the twentieth century. Today most middle and even low-income nations have formal employment-based retirement systems, although many of those remain seriously inadequate. In this chapter we focus on the sources of retirement security among older individuals in Latin America, with a particular focus on Mexico. Mexico introduced an employment-based defined-benefit retirement scheme in 1943. That system was plagued by numerous problems, and even after radical reforms, including a switch to private defined-contribution plans, problems of labor force informality, low contribution densities, and low replacement rates persist. As a result, Mexico, like many other nations, has introduced state and federal noncontributory pensions, upon which most older individuals rely. Although these pensions address

http://dx.doi.org/10.1891/0198-8794.40.127

the immediate problem of extreme poverty among older persons, they are minimal and reintroduce the long-term problems of fiscal unsustainability. We discuss the growing role of civil society organizations (CSOs) in advocating for the social and human rights of older persons.

INTRODUCTION

In the United States Social Security significantly reduced poverty among older individuals (Engelhardt & Gruber, 2004). Before passage of the program old age was a period of serious economic vulnerability for older citizens. Along with access to healthcare, old age economic security represents a core component of the modern welfare state. We trace its beginning to conservative Prussian Chancellor Otto von Bismarck, who, after the consolidation of Germany in the 19th century, introduced old-age economic security, disability coverage, and more to counter the appeal of Marxism among the working classes (Hennock, 2007). Subsequently, all high and middle-income nations introduced some form of retirement income system, usually funded by contributions from employees and employers. Such programs are extremely expensive, especially as they mature, and the reality is that many nations simply cannot afford them. In many developing nations, even after the introduction of employment-based retirement plans, serious poverty among older individuals persisted and other solutions needed to be found.

In this chapter we briefly review the shortcomings of the original pension systems in Latin America and the nature and consequences of the reforms that were attempted. In most countries in the region, high levels of labor force informality and inadequate contributions meant that both defined-benefit schemes and the privatized defined-contribution plans that replaced them could not guarantee an adequate income in old age. Given the inability of even the most drastic reforms to guarantee minimally adequate retirement income, many nations have introduced noncontributory pensions to address the serious economic vulnerability of older citizens. We focus specifically on Mexico, a middle-income nation with a rapidly aging population. Other authors in this volume address the specifics of pension and retirement systems in detail so we will not do so in this chapter, other than to emphasize the unique problems that plague such systems in nations like Mexico. We also introduce the issue of the role of civil society organizations in the struggle for the economic rights of older persons. This struggle, as we discuss, takes place within a broader struggle for human rights generally, and the human and social rights of older persons more specifically. As part of this new discourse social rights are framed as central to the meaningful exercise of human rights.

Latin America is unique in the extent to which a series of international conventions has codified the human and social rights of older persons. Such conventions clearly signal a change in the discourse related to aging and the capacities and rights of older citizens. These conventions and the debates surrounding them reflect a change in the portrayal of old age as a period in which one loses one's autonomy and becomes dependent to one of "active aging" and "active citizenship," in which old age is framed as a productive and engaged period of life in which one's autonomy remains as intact as possible. The question that remains is whether and how such conventions translate into effective national and local legislation and practice, especially in nations with limited resources that face major fiscal crises related to the support of rapidly aging populations. It is in that context that the possibilities of civil society take on special significance.

Pensions in Latin America

Latin American nations began introducing social insurance programs in the 1920s and 1930s (Mesa-Lago, 2008). Argentina, Brazil, Chile, Costa Rica, Cuba, and Uruguay introduced their programs early, beginning in the 1920s. Mexico, along with Bolivia, Colombia, Ecuador, Panama, Peru, and Venezuela introduced pension systems in the 1940s and 1950s. Other Latin American nations followed. As in most other cases, Mexico introduced a defined-benefit, employment-based, pay-as-you go pension system. In general, when such schemes are first introduced their program costs are manageable since there are many active workers contributing to the plan relative to the number of retirees. As such plans mature and as social changes reduce the size of the active labor force and as life expectancies increase, they face serious long-term fiscal crises (Orenstein, 2008, 2011).

In most nations of Latin America, pension systems suffered from serious problems related to low rates of coverage, low contribution densities, gender inequities, and low income replacement rates (Barrientos, 1998; Madrid, 2003). Their major weakness, though, has continued to result from the fact that they cover only formal sector workers. In Mexico over half of workers are employed in the informal sector, where they lack contracts and do not pay into the Social Security system (Aguila, López-Ortega, & Gutiérrez Robledo, 2018). During their working years many workers move back and forth between formal and informal employment and often contribute only for a few years (International Labour Organization [ILO], 2019; Maloney, 2004). Since they lack private retirement plans, a large fraction of the population continues to work well into old age (Aguila, Díaz, Fu, Kapteyn, & Pierson, 2011). Even after the fairly drastic structural reforms that have been introduced in recent years, principally in the form of a move to privatized individual defined-contribution plans, the long-term outlook for pension systems in most of Latin America remains bleak (Alonso, Hoyo,

& Tuesta, 2015; Torre & Rudolph, 2018). In this context, one of the major objectives of civil society organizations is to attempt to guarantee at least a minimal income to older individuals who do not qualify for Social Security.

Defamilisation: Social Policy and Older People

The term "defamilisation" is used to refer to the shift in responsibility for social support from the family to the state. Nations differ greatly in the extent to which official social policy reflects defamilisation. In the conservative welfare states of central and southern Europe, social policy continues to focus on the family, whereas in the more social democratic nations of northern Europe, the state assumes many of those support functions (Esping-Andersen, 1990; Palier, 2010). We place Latin American nations squarely in the highly familistic category. For the most part, family support policies in those countries are based on a traditional gender-based male-breadwinner model (Becker, 1981; Esping-Andersen, 1990; Horrell & Humphries, 1997). In previous eras this arrangement may have allowed the family to address its own social support needs, but times and circumstances have changed.

In posttraditional societies, which increasingly include the nations of central and southern Europe as well as the nations of Latin America, the male-breadwinner model no longer functions. Extensive social changes including smaller families, migration, increasing divorce rates, the need for women to work, and greatly increased life spans means that the family can no longer assume the full responsibility for aging parents. Increasingly, the state assumes greater responsibility for the support and care of older citizens (Esping-Andersen, 1996; Michoń, 2008).

In contrast to defamilisation, the term "refamilisation" refers to attempts to reaffirm the family's role. The family and social policies of the conservative corporatist nations of central and southern Europe continue to reaffirm the role of the family in the care of aging parents and others, even as the family and its support functions are evolving in ways that make such policies seriously obsolete (Palier, 2010). As we discuss in the following, Latin American conventions related to the human and social rights of older persons reaffirm family support as a basic right. Such conservative policies are particularly resistant to significant change even as it becomes clear that they fail to address the emerging reality (Esping-Andrsen, 2010; Palier, 2010). Although defamilisation remains far less pronounced in Latin America and other developing regions than in higher-income nations, even there, noncontributory pensions and other public services are becoming more important as the family's ability to support and care for aging parents is reduced by the same social changes that have so profoundly affected the developed world.

The Changing Welfare State and Older Citizens

Healthcare and old-age security continue to be the most central and costliest protections that the state provides its citizens. Given the rapid aging of the populations of most nations, the fiscal burden on the state is huge and growing. The responses by governments have been shaped by the ways in which the sources of the problem are framed. Christine Lagarde, Managing Director of the International Monetary Fund, and others see the problem as primarily one of demographics and increasing life spans (Hutchens, 2016). From this perspective, the dramatic increase in the proportion of older individuals relative to those of working age creates a dependency burden that is unsustainable. According to José Piñera, a neoliberal economist who was central to the expansion of privatized pensions in developing countries and who served as Chilean Secretary of Labor and Social Security from 1978 to 1980 under President Augusto Pinochet, the burden of traditional pay-as-you-go retirement plans will inevitably result in resentment among younger workers who will be forced to contribute an ever growing fraction of their earnings to the support of retired workers (Piñera, Fall/Winter 1995/96). Such arrangements clearly seem unsustainable. Indeed, it is hard to imagine that there is not a limit to the burden one can place on the active labor force. Regardless of one's political position, some other solution must be found. Given the dominance of neoliberal social policies, a radical redistribution of wealth in any country seems unlikely. So far, most reforms have made rather modest changes to existing systems.

To date, the most radical reforms of pension systems have involved their privatization, a solution that rejects the original solidaristic principle on which traditional retirement income schemes were based (Arrizabalo Montoro, del Rosal, & Javier Murillo Arroyo, 2019; McCarthy, 2017). Many developing countries, including most Latin American nations, have adopted some version of this defined-contribution approach (Arza, 2012; Madrid, 2003; Mesa-Lago, 2004, 2008), although many have modified their initial plans to deal with a wide range of problems inherent in such schemes, primarily related to low contribution and savings levels. Argentina abandoned the experiment altogether and returned to a fully defined-benefit arrangement. Despite initial hopes that privatized retirement schemes would increase savings and foster economic development, the results were largely disappointing. Even as late as 2000 only 22% of the Mexican labor force was covered (Willmore, 2014).

For many critics of defined-contribution approaches, primarily from the left, the source of the problem results from an unjust and inequitable distribution of wealth and status in society at large. Forcing workers to finance their own retirement security through potentially volatile and risky investments only makes matters worse. Given the insurmountable problem of incomplete employment coverage many nations have introduced a minimal guaranteed income to individuals who do not have access to a formal pension. Such pensions clearly address problems of extreme inequity and poverty, but they reintroduce the dilemma of long-term fiscal sustainability (Aguila, Mejia, Perez-Arce, Ramirez, & Rivera Illingworth, 2016).

Pension Reform, Solidarity, and Noncontributory Pensions

Traditional defined-benefit pay-as-you-go retirement systems, if they are sufficiently inclusive, institutionalize an intergenerational bond of solidarity as younger workers directly support older retirees in the expectation that they, in turn, will be supported by future generations. Such social bonds reproduce the expectation that adult children contribute to the care and support of their aging parents. In reality, though, low participation rates in developing countries, including those of Latin America, probably limited the social solidaristic potential of many schemes. Whatever solidaristic potential existed in the old defined-benefit system, though, was forfeited by the switch to fully funded individual investment plans. Such a transition redefines solidarity from a tie between generations to a tie between one's younger self and one's older self. The structural connection between generations inherent in older pension systems is severed.

Although privatized pension plans address the long-term fiscal crises of pension systems, they do so at a potentially high social cost. In addition to a loss of whatever bond of solidarity traditional pay-as-you-go systems fostered, without other reforms these plans could not address problems of incomplete coverage, gender inequity, episodic contribution, and inadequate retirement income. To address the problem of seriously incomplete coverage, Latin American countries, including Mexico, have introduced various forms of noncontributory pensions or adopted more flexible rules for qualification for state pensions (Barrientos, 2012; Rofman, Apella, & Vezza, 2013). Such noncontributory pensions have become the main source of income security for older individuals in at least 40 countries around the world (Newson & Bourne, 2011; Willmore, 2006).

In Mexico noncontributory pensions have made pension coverage nearly universal (Willmore, 2014). Without such pensions most Mexican workers would receive nothing. In 2019 only 23% of women and 40% of men had access to a contributory pension (Secretaría de Bienestar, 2019). Making matters worse, fully 26% of older adults had neither a pension nor access to public programs. In response to this vulnerability, noncontributory pensions were initially provided by local governments, beginning with Mexico City in 2001. In 2007 the federal government introduced a noncontributory pension program named "Setenta y Mas" (70 and older) for adults 70 or older living in rural areas with less than 2,500 inhabitants. This program was expanded to all localities with fewer than

20,000 inhabitants in 2008, and to all places with fewer than 30,000 inhabitants in 2009. In 2012 it was extended to all older persons not receiving any other Social Security benefits or state-level noncontributory pensions (Aguila et al., 2018). Currently the program, which is referred to as the *Programa Pensión para Adultos Mayores* (Pension Program for Older Adults), covers individuals 65 and older who live in indigenous communities and certain individuals registered as special rights holders in the program, and those 68 and older in the rest of the country (Secretaría de Bienestar, 2019). In 2019 recipients received $1,275 pesos (US$64.87) per month paid bimonthly.

Currently, most older adults in Mexico rely on these state or federal noncontributory pensions, which are significantly smaller than Social Security benefits (Aguila et al., 2018). Although these programs have greatly reduced the number of older individuals with no income, the level of support is minimal and a large fraction of Mexican elders live in poverty and many continue to work after 65 (Aguila et al., 2011). In addition, as we have noted, the reliance on public funding reintroduces the long-term fiscal risks for national economies that older pay-as-you-go pension systems involved (Filgueira & Manzi, 2017). Yet in light of the growing number of individuals with little income, few resources, and no retirement plan, these basic pensions are an essential lifeline. For that reason, they are a major focus of civil society efforts, which work to ensure that older individuals who are entitled to benefits in fact receive them.

Like other government support programs once they are introduced, noncontributory pensions develop an inertia of their own and individuals resist losing them or having their payment levels reduced. Interviews with civil society activists makes the importance of a basic pension clear, and also the extent to which individuals are willing to go to protect them. Much of the community action of civil society organizers in Mexico involves motivating elders to demand their right to a minimal pension, in addition to assisting them overcome the administrative hurdles to qualifying. What is clear is that the struggle for a basic pension draws these organizations' attention to other areas of need and motivates older group members to engage in political action. Such activities foster an immediate form of direct democracy that empowers individuals to act to further their own interests and the social and human rights of older people in general. Although states must deal with fiscal realities, experiments with neoliberalism and an excessive focus on the market and economic issues alone ignores essential social realities and place equity and full citizenship behind profit.

Before proceeding to a discussion of the various conventions and statements that comprise the body of soft law related to the new discourse on the rights of older persons, it would be useful to review the ways in which the problem is framed, by which we mean the ways in which the problem is defined and appropriate solutions presented as legitimate and effective. Although biological aging may be an objective fact, the situation of older persons, including their rights and obligations, are social constructions. Older people can be viewed as superannuated and unproductive, or they can be seen as autonomous agents who are not only potentially productive and able to care for themselves, but entirely capable of contributing significantly to the common good.

"Frame analysis" and "frame alignment processes," refer to ways in which social movements or groups convince a larger audience that their interpretation of some situation is accurate and that their proposed solutions are both just and likely to be effective (Goffman, 1974; Snow, Burke Rochford, Worden, & Benford, 1986). The basic process involves changing the public's interpretation of some situation as accidental, unavoidable, or inevitable to seeing it as the result of injustice (Turner, 1969). Rather than simple charity or compassion, the new interpretation requires the elimination of the injustice. This approach complements and adds a new dimension to resource mobilization theory, which focuses on the economic, political, and social resources that a group has at its disposal that it can bring to bear in furthering its cause by reintroducing cultural and cognitive understandings to the very practical focus on resources and capacities alone.

"Master frames" refer to widely held understandings of the causes of a particular situation, including the ways in which it can be altered. These are more general than specific frames focused on a specific issue. Takeshi Wada presents quantitative data to argue that during the neoliberal period in Mexico, earlier claims for social rights took on a new aspect as demands for political rights, which are basic to gaining civil and social rights (Wada, 2006). Rita Noonan argues that women were able to protest in Pinochet's Chile in ways that men were not because they could use a master frame of motherhood and femininity to protest human rights abuses since the focus on womanhood was compatible with the regime's own master frame of veneration of the home and family (Noonan, 1995). While resource mobilization theory's focus on the material capacity and skills necessary for successful protest, frame analysis adds a focus on peoples' and groups' understandings and the deliberate and strategic actions they take to attempt to change perceptions in order to address a particular injustice.

In the case of older people, society can either treat them as the victims of misfortune or unavoidable aging processes, or treat them more as possessing autonomy and basic rights. This involves reframing public perceptions of older persons as weak and helpless to recognizing their very real productive potential and respecting their agency and autonomy. In the first frame, the solution is compassion and charity; in the second, it involves advocacy and efforts to change the basic rules of the game that disadvantage certain segments of the elderly population. As a culmination of a long series of international conventions and statements on the rights of older persons, in 2015 the Inter-American Convention for the Protection of the Human Rights of Older Persons (IACPHROP) issued a major report which affirmed the right of older persons to social participation, as well as political participation and nondiscrimination (Organization of American States [OAS], 2015a). The right to participation is held to be central to the protection of other human rights. Theoretically and practically, then, the question that the report leads us to pose is how civil society organizations mobilize citizens and help to create social and political environments in which they can act as effective agents in furthering their own interests and those of others.

The Human and Social Rights of Older People: Beyond Demography
During the latter half of the 20th century demographers developed a theory that relates historical changes in fertility and mortality to overall population size (Kirk, 1996). Demographic transition theory proposed four stages in the transition of human populations from primitive to modern profiles. Stage 1 refers to the period before industrialization and improvements in agricultural production that was characterized by high fertility and high mortality that resulted in a small, but stable population. In Stage 2, as conditions of life improved, mortality rates began to decline while fertility rates remained high, resulting in a rapid increase in population. In Stage 3, as people expected their children to survive, fertility rates began to decline, even as mortality rates continued to drop, resulting in slightly slower population growth. In Stage 4, both fertility and mortality both reach low levels and the population again remains stable, if much larger than at the beginning of this process.

Demographic transition theory is useful in drawing attention to the impact of technological and social changes on population size and composition and also for making the point that different population age profiles call for different policy and social responses. A young population has different needs for education, healthcare, economic support, and much more than a population that is much older, and it is likely that in the two cases the dominant public policies will be quite different. Whether the demographic transition process holds in all of its details for all nations or regions remains disputed (Nielsen, 2015; Zaidi & Morgan, 2017), but it need not be strictly true in every detail to be useful for our purposes. Whatever the details or exact sequence of events, the aging of the populations of the world is hardly in dispute.

In recent years some observers have proposed a fifth stage to this demographic transition, again one that implies significant cultural and political adjustment that are relevant to our discussion. This new fifth stage refers to a period when fertility rates drop below mortality rates. Mathematically, such a situation eventually leads to population decline and the sort of rapid population aging we have been discussing. Today, birth rates in Europe are below replace-ment, as they are in 15 countries in Latin America (Eurostat, 2019; Montes-de-Oca, Paredes, Rodríguez, & Garay, 2018). In order to replace herself and one male a woman must bear 2.1 or more children. The fraction is to compensate for some unavoidable loss. Maintaining a stable population requires replenish-ment from somewhere. Even though Germany's fertility rate is below replace-ment, it continues to grow as the result of immigration (World Economic Forum, 2019). Europe and much of the rest of the developed world are facing serious dilemmas resulting from their need for immigrants and growing anti-immigrant sentiments.

But our objective does not directly relate to immigration. Rather, our point is that the arrival of the fifth stage in the demographic transition brings with it a shift in policy discourse from one focused solely on the needs of younger groups to a greater focus on the welfare and needs of older persons and what they are able to contribute to the community wealth. A major focus of that new dis-course relates to the human and social rights of older persons (Choi, Brownell, & Moldovan, 2017; Martin, Rodríguez, & Brown, 2015; Montes-de-Oca et al., 2018; OAS, 2015a, 2017; Rodriguez-Pinzón & Martin, 2003). This focus on rights, in addition to the material and psychological well-being of older persons, is rather recent and definitely in a process of evolution.

The issue of the human and social rights of older persons may at first sight seem uncomplicated. After all, major international conventions, such as the Universal Declaration of Human Rights, adopted by the United Nations General Assembly in 1948 (United Nations, 1948) and later conventions affirm that all humans are entitled to basic rights. Unfortunately, until recently none of these conventions identified older people as a group whose rights require special pro-tection. Affirmations of general human rights are useful, but groups with special needs can be overlooked if they are not singled out. More recent conventions, particularly in Latin America, have addressed this omission, at least in principle. The question we are left with is the extent to which this new focus on the rights of older persons is accompanied by real improvements in the situation of older persons.

In their recent review of international and regional law related to the rights of older persons, Martin, Rodríguez, and Pinzón differentiate between what they term "soft" law and "hard" law related to the rights of older people (Martin et al., 2015). Soft law, which we might really think of as principles rather than law, includes statements such as those expressed in the United Nations Madrid International Plan of Action on Aging (MIPAA) which sets out general principles related to the rights of older people (United Nations, 1948). Such principles are not binding nor enforceable in any legal system (del Toro Huerta, 2006). Hard law, on the other hand, refers to national or more local laws, which are often informed by international law, that are at some level binding. Soft law is couched in terms of general strategies or approaches which may eventually become what the authors term "customary law," which is still not enforceable, but which reflect a greater acceptance of the underlying obligations. Soft laws, or the codification of principles that affirm human rights in principle, are useful in changing discourses, but their real success is reflected in more binding legislation.

An example of how soft law can reify principles to the point that they become customary law, for which there are more mechanisms for monitoring nations' compliance, is the Inter-American Convention of Protecting the Human Rights of Older Persons approved in June 2015 by the Organization of American States (Montes-de-Oca et al., 2018). States that ratify the convention agree to abide by its principles. In order to monitor implementation and compliance the Convention includes a follow-up mechanism consisting of a Conference of States Parties and a Committee of Experts who are charged with the monitoring task (OAS, 2015b). Of course, there is no real enforcement mechanism and guaranteeing compliance in effect involves moral suasion, and the fact that signatory nations agree to allow their policies and practices related to the rights of older persons to be made public. Currently five countries, Argentina, Bolivia, Chile, Costa Rica, and Uruguay, have ratified the convention.

Latin America has made particularly impressive strides in codifying and affirming the human rights of older persons. The extent to which these conventions have resulted in actual improvements in the situation of older individuals, and especially those with special needs and few resources, remains unclear (Sidorenko & Zaidi, 2018). Few of these new conventions represent hard law. Certain of the principles upheld are little more than affirmations of traditional approaches, such as statements that older people have a right to family support

The Human Rights Debate

Before proceeding, though, we must point out that the concept of human rights is not a universally accepted or valued concept, nor is it clear that the global struggle for human rights is even close to being won. The current rise in populist nationalism in so many parts of the world is frankly disconcerting (Jeppesen, 2016; Strangio, 2017). More than 70 years after the adoption of the Universal Declaration of Human Rights, many human rights activists, including Amnesty International's Secretary-General, Salil Shetty, have serious concerns regarding real progress and the possibility of retreat in many places (Hopgood, 2013; Posner, 2014; Sikkink, 2017). Treaties and conventions codify principles, but their adoption in law, and especially the enforcement of real protections by local governments, is not guaranteed by any international body.

David Kennedy, a human rights activist himself, offers a detailed summary of criticisms of legal conceptions of human rights that have been leveled over the years (Kennedy, 2002).

We will not delve into these except to note that among the most serious criticisms is that traditional human rights claims represented little more than an imposition of Western cultural values on others (García, Klare, & Williams, 2015; Hopgood, 2013; Kennedy, 2002; Moyn, 2010; Tharoor, 1999/2000). Westerners may privilege the individual and view their autonomy and agency as paramount, but other cultures may privilege the will of the group, clan, or tribe over that of the individual. In the absence of a native's understanding of local values and customs, the imposition of ethical concepts, no matter how dearly held by an outsider, could end up doing more harm than good in terms of the well-being of locals. Certain observers have basically given up the hope of extending full human rights to all currently excluded or stigmatized groups. It is important to note, though, that the Human Rights Movement has become far more sensitive to cultural and local differences. Recent efforts at understanding and fostering human rights take cultural differences, gender, and other important distinctions seriously (García et al., 2015).

Kathryn Sikkink defends the utility and basic success of efforts to extend and strengthen human rights (Sikkink, 2017). While increases in the number of refugees, and local atrocities, such as those in the Democratic Republic of the Congo or Bosnia, can temper one's optimism, overall Sikkink notes substantial progress in women's rights, the abolition of capital punishment, and more. She offers a plausible explanation for the appearance of a lack of progress when she points out that furthering the agenda entails drawing attention to human rights abuses, a framing tactic that can make it appear that little progress is being made, when in fact the exposure of such abuses affirms the success of the effort. Today, human rights abuses can no longer remain hidden, and governments can no longer violate human rights with impunity as they could just a few years ago (Keck & Sikkink, 1998).

From our perspective, an appreciation of cultural differences does not preclude general affirmations of universal basic principles related to the human and social rights of older persons as they are affirmed in the conventions we discuss in the following. In addition, although progress may be slow, the only alternative to a forceful affirmation and defense of basic rights is despair and acceptance of the status quo, a position that is unacceptable. Additionally, we are less interested in the imposition of external conceptions of human and social rights on specific groups. Rather we are more interested in the ways in which local groups define their own agendas and the ways in which they frame the issues they address. Local groups may well be influenced by national and even international social movements and ideas, but they must be implemented at a local level by individuals working in voluntary groups.

The Evolution of an Agenda

Advocacy for human and social rights has a long history in Latin America (Sikkink, 2017). The 1917 Mexican constitution was the first constitution in the world to affirm economic and social rights. The history of dictatorships and violence in the region might overshadow this reality, but human and social rights have been a core concern, at least in principle, in Latin America. The history of dictatorships in the region clearly have forced the issue into public discourse. We trace the beginning of the contemporary discourse on the human and social rights of older persons to the Report of the World Assembly on Aging, which met in Vienna, Austria from July 26 to August 6, 1982 in the first international convention intended to provide guiding principles that nations could follow in addressing the needs of growing elderly populations (United Nations, 1982). It was preceded by various UN statements on the rights of older persons, but Vienna represented the first modern attempt to comprehensively address the issue. The assembly offered 62 recommendations for action to further research, data collection and analysis, training and education of healthcare providers, and more. The recommendations dealt with health and nutrition, the protection of elderly consumers, housing and environment, family, social welfare, income security and employment, and education (United Nations, 1982).

Monitoring and assessing the impact of such international recommendations and principles at the national and more local levels proved difficult and periodic assessments of the situation of older persons in various nations revealed disappointing progress toward the Assembly's goals. Low levels of economic development, political upheavals, recessions, and other factors undermined the implementation of the proposals (Sidorenko & Zaidi, 2018). The limited results of the Vienna Assembly led to renewed efforts by the Second World Assembly on Aging (SWAA), which produced the MIPAA (Montes-de-Oca et al., 2018). The Madrid conference framed the situation of aging populations as one that goes beyond issues of demography and population composition to one involving the human and social rights of older persons (United Nations, 2002). Point 4 of the introduction of the Assembly's report states that "[p]opulation ageing is poised to become a major issue in developing countries, which are projected to age swiftly in the first half of the twenty-first century. The proportion of older persons is expected to rise from 8 to 19 per cent by 2050, while that of children will fall from 33 to 22 per cent" (p. 5). The report details unique vulnerabilities associated with gender, rural residence, and more. It calls for "...changes in attitudes, policies and practices at all levels in all sectors so that the enormous potential of ageing in the twenty-first century may be fulfilled" (p. 7). Accomplishing this would require an international effort and consciousness raising at all levels of government and society.

In the days before SWAA, civil society organizations held a forum of their own to affirm the dignity of age and further the agenda on the basic rights of older people (Montes-de-Oca et al., 2018). Their efforts included collaborations with academics, government institutions, businesses, and others to begin to build a social movement. These multilateral and civil society initiatives have been carried forward with particular success in Latin America where successive regional and intergovernmental meetings have developed general principles and public policy applicable to the region. These included the Regional Strategy for the Implementation in Latin America and the Caribbean of the MIPAA meetings in Santiago de Chile in 2003; Brasilia, Brazil in 2007; San José, Costa Rica in 2012; and Asunción, Paraguay in 2017. Each iteration reaffirmed and refined the basic agenda. In parallel, civil society organizations representing older persons met to produce several declarations. These took place in Santiago de Chile in 2003; in Brasilia in 2007; in Tres Ríos, Costa Rica in 2012; and in Ypacaraí, Paraguay in 2017. During this period the Montevideo Consensus on Population and Development (MCPD) drafted in 2013 and the IACPHROP drafted by the Organization of American States in 2015 further affirmed the rights agenda. The sequence of these meetings is summarized in Figure 6.1 (Montes-de-Oca et al., 2018).

These various conferences and meetings of governmental representatives and civil society organizations are clearly important in furthering the rights dialogue related to older persons. The 2017 Asunción Declaration, with the subtitle "Building Inclusive Societies: Ageing with Dignity and Rights" summarizes the spirit of these efforts. It consists of 22 propositions and affirmations and general objectives. The following four serve as examples:

1. Reaffirm the commitment of our Governments to promote, protect and respect the human rights, dignity and fundamental freedoms of all older persons, without discrimination of any kind, and ratify the responsibility of States to ensure ageing with dignity and rights, with the greatest possible quality of life and full enjoyment of the rights of older persons;

3. Reiterate that the San José Charter on the Rights of Older Persons in Latin America and the Caribbean offers a regional framework for public policymaking that States continue to adopt, that complements the work of other mechanisms at the regional and international levels, and that helps to strengthen protection of the human rights and fundamental freedoms of older persons;

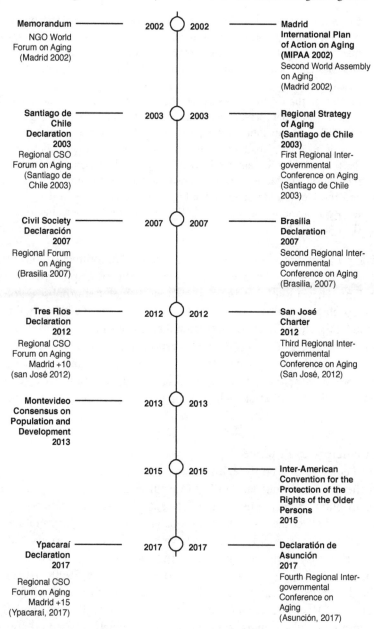

FIGURE 6.1 Timeline of regional and intergovernmental meetings 2002–2017. CSO, civil society organizations.

Source: Data from Montes-de-Oca, V., Paredes, M., Vicente Rodríguez, & Garay, S. (2018). Older persons and human rights in Latin America and the Caribbean. *International Journal on Ageing in Developing Countries,* 2(2), 149–164. Retrieved from https://www.inia.org.mt/wp-content/uploads/2018/09/2.2-8-Montes-de-Oca-edited.pdf

5. Urge the Governments to build the issue of ageing into their development policies, plans and programmes in a cross-cutting manner, and to implement specific policies for older persons that recognize gender inequalities and promote their autonomy and independence, as well as intergenerational solidarity...

12. Encourage the Governments of the region to consider the situation and interests of older persons, including also the ethnicity, race, gender, disability and generational perspectives, in the design and implementation of national plans and programmes to promote achievement of the 2030 Agenda for Sustainable Development and the Sustainable Development Goals, the Montevideo Consensus on Population and Development, and the Montevideo Strategy for Implementation of the Regional Gender Agenda within the Sustainable Development Framework by 2030.... (ECLAC, 2017)

The propositions all begin with terms such as "Recommend," "Call upon," "Urge," and "Request," terms which emphasize the principled nature of the propositions. They are soft law in the sense that they do not propose enforceable edicts or specific programs. They serve as policy guidance to individual nations which must take their local and subnational situations into account in applying the general principles. The longer-term questions relate to the responsiveness of governments in adopting policies favorable to the human and social rights of older persons, and the extent to which civil society organizations have been effective in forcing the adoption of such policies.

From Principle to Practice

As Martin et al. note, even though soft laws do not have the force of the courts behind them, they do not lack utility (Martin et al., 2015). They can lead to changes in public perceptions, redefine acceptable discourse concerning aging and rights, and affect the visibility of various groups. Although several new laws that affirm the rights of older persons have been passed in various nations in Latin America, they have been difficult to put into practice. Laws related to the rights of older persons have been introduced since the early 1990s (Huenchuan, 2013) and have been reinforced by institutional commitments and structures (Huenchuan, 2016). The specific objectives of these laws differ substantially, and many continue to affirm an assistance perspective which is based on conceptualizations of those over a certain age as unproductive and in need of care and assistance (Huenchuan, 2016). More recent laws have begun affirming a rights perspective, which includes the right to a dignified life; a dignified death; equality and nondiscrimination; physical, psychological, and emotional autonomy; and the right to participate in the social, cultural, and political life of the community (Huenchuan, 2013). These principles and rights were fully consolidated in the IACPHROP (OAS, 2015a).

In Mexico, a number of laws dealing with the welfare of older adults have been introduced at the national and subnational levels. These largely reaffirm the family's responsibility for aging parents, while extending and standardizing the provision of diverse services and assistance. Today the family continues to provide most of the care and support that older parents receive (Montes de Oca Zavala, 2014). That responsibility is codified in the National Law on the Rights of older persons, Article 9 (Cámara De Diputados Del H. Congreso De La Unión (Mexico), 2018, p. 7). Without minimizing the significant advance that this law represents in affirming the rights of older persons, we must note that it does not specifically address the rights of older ethnic group members, nor does it deal directly with economic security or pensions. Rather, it reaffirms the right to social assistance and the right to be supported by the family, rather than affirming the right to a public pension or support. Despite its shortcomings, though, this reform strengthens subnational laws and constitutes a substantial move forward in the reframing of the justification for social programs and public policies focused on older persons as possessing basic social rights. It is important to note that these basic principles were again reaffirmed at the Fourth Regional Intergovernmental Conference on aging and the rights of older persons held in Asunción, Paraguay in 2017 (CEPAL, 2017).

CONCLUSION

Greatly extended life spans, the fiscal crisis of the state, in conjunction with demographic and social changes to the family that reduce its ability to provide all of the support and care aging parents need, require new ways of addressing the economic and social vulnerability of older citizens, especially in middle-income nations like Mexico. As we have discussed, traditional and even drastically reformed employment-based retirement income schemes proved to be seriously inadequate and in Mexico covered only a small fraction of the working-age population. As a result, many individuals are forced to work well into old age and many suffer serious poverty.

Civil society organizations and other activists have been instrumental in demanding protecting and furthering the human and social rights of older individuals (Angel, Montes de Oca, & Rodríguez, 2018). A core objective has been to force the state to introduce noncontributory pensions to address the serious shortcomings of the employment-based retirement schemes. Although these noncontributory pensions are tiny, they provide some basic income security and protection against grinding poverty. Unfortunately, like older pay-as-you-go retirement systems noncontributory pensions reintroduce a major fiscal burden for local, state, and national governments. As Mexico's population continues to age this problem will become ever more serious and efforts to protect basic income supports for vulnerable old people will represent a major challenge for civil society organizations, including those organized by older people themselves. Today, the number of such organizations is growing rapidly and existing non-governmental organizations are extending their missions to include issues related to advocacy for and service provision to older citizens. Their role is evolving and given the level of need, it is likely to expand.

REFERENCES

Aguila, E., Díaz, C., Fu, M. M., Kapteyn, A., & Pierson, A. (2011). *Living longer in Mexico: Income security and health.* Washington, DC: AARP.

Aguila, E., López-Ortega, M., & Gutiérrez Robledo, L. M. (2018). Non-contributory pension programs and frailty of older adults: Evidence from Mexico. *PLOS ONE*, 13(11). https://doi.org/10.1371/journal.pone.0206792

Aguila, E., Mejia, N., Perez-Arce, F., Ramirez, E., & Rivera Illingworth, A. (2016). Costs of extending the noncontributory pension program for elderly: The Mexican case. *Journal of Aging & Social Policy*, 28(4), 325–343. http://dx.doi.org/10.1080/08959420.2016.1158384

Alonso, J., Hoyo, C., & Tuesta, D. (2015). A model for the pension system in Mexico: Diagnosis and recommendations. *Journal of Pension Economics and Finance*, 14(1), 76–112. http://dx.doi.org/10.1017/S147474721400016X

Arrizabalo, Montoro, X., del Rosal, M., & Javier Murillo Arroyo, F. (2019). The debate on pension systems: The paradigmatic cases of Chile and Spain. *American Journal of Economics and Sociology*, 78(1), 195–223. http://dx.doi.org/10.1111/ajes.12262

Arza, C. (2012). Basic old-age protection in Latin America: Noncontributory pensions, coverage expansion strategies, and aging patterns across countries. *Population and Development Review*, S46–S60. http://dx.doi.org/10.1111/padr.12267

Angel, R., Montes de Oca, V., & Rodríguez, V. (2018). Strengthened solidarity: A theoretical inquiry into the role of civil society organizations in the support of elderly citizens in Mexico City. In W. Vega, J. Angel, L. M. Gutiérrez, & K. Markides, *Contextualizing health and aging in the Americas* (pp. 159–180). Springer. https://doi.org/10.1007/978-3-030-00584-9_8

Barrientos, A. (1998). *Pension reform in Latin America.* Aldershot, England: Ashgate.

Barrientos, A. (2012). Dilemas de las politicas sociales latinoamericanas. ¿Hacia una protección social fragmentada? *Nueva Sociedad*, 239, 65–78. Retrieved from https://nuso.org/media/articles/downloads/3847_1.pdf

Becker, G. S. (1981). *A treatise on the family*. Cambridge, MA: Harvard University Press.

Cámara De Diputados Del, H. Congreso De La Uníon (Mexico). (2018). Ley de Los Derechos de Las personas adultas mayores. In S. G. d. S. Parlamentarios (Ed.), *Nueva ley publicada en el diario oficial de la federación el 25 de junio de 2018*. Retrieved from http://www.diputados.gob.mx/LeyesBiblio/pdf/245_120718.pdf

CEPAL. (2017). *Derechos de las persona mayores: Retos para la interdependencia y autonomía*. Santiago, Chile: Natione Unidas: Comisión Económica para América Latina y el Caribe (CEPAL). Retrieved from https://www.cepal.org/es/publicaciones/41471-derechos-personas-mayores-retos-la-interdependencia-autonomia

Choi, M., Brownell, P., & Moldovan, S. I. (2017). International movement to promote human rights of older women with a focus on violence and abuse against older women. *International Social Work, 60*(1), 170–181. http://dx.doi.org/10.1177/0020872814559562

del Toro Huerta, M. I. (2006). El fenómeno del soft law y las nuevas perspectivas del derecho internacional. *Anuario Mexicano de Derecho Internacional, 6*, 513–549. Distrito Federal, México: Universidad Nacional Autónoma de México. http://dx.doi.org/10.22201/iij.24487872e.2006.6.160

ECLAC. (2017). *Asunción declaration building inclusive societies: Ageing with dignity and rights*. Fourth Regional Intergovernmental Conference on Ageing and the Rights of Older Persons in Latin America and the Caribbean. Retrieved from https://conferenciaenvejecimiento.cepal.org/4/sites/envejecimiento4/files/c1700061 4_0.pdf

Engelhardt, G. V., & Gruber, J. (2004). *Social security and the evolution of elderly poverty*. National Bureau of Economic Research. Working Paper 10466. Cambridge, MA. Retrieved from https://www.nber.org/papers/w10466.pdf.

Esping-Andersen, G. (1990). *The three worlds of welfare capitalism*. Princeton, NJ: Princeton University Press.

Esping-Andersen, G. (1996). Welfare states without work: The impasse of labor shedding and familialism in continental European social policy. In G. Esping-Andersen (Ed.), *Welfare states in transition: National adaptations in global economics* (pp. 66–87). Thousand Oaks, CA: Sage.

Esping-Andrsen, G. (2010). Prologue: What does it mean to break with Bismarck? In B. Palier (Ed.), *A long goodbye to Bismarck? The politics of welfare reform in continental Europe* (pp. 13–18). Amsterdam, the Netherlands: Amsterdam University Press.

Eurostat. (2019). *Fertility statistics*. Retrieved from https://ec.europa.eu/eurostat/statistics-explained/index.php/Fertility_statistics

Filgueira, F., & Manzi, P. (2017). *Pension and income transfers for old age Inter- and intragenerational distribution in comparative perspective*. Retrieved from http://repositorio .cepal.org/bitstream/handle/11362/42087/1/S1700520_en.pdf. In: United Nation (ECLAC)

García, H. A., Klare, K., & Williams, L. A (Eds.). (2015). *Social and economic rights in theory and practice*. New York, NY: Routledge.

Goffman, E. (1974). *Frame analysis*. Cambridge, MA: Harvard University Press.

Hennock, E. P. (2007). *The origin of the welfare state in England and Germany, 1850-1914: Social policies compared*. Cambridge, UK: Cambridge University Press.

Hopgood, S. (2013). *The endtimes of human rights*. Ithaca, NY: Cornell University Press.

Horrell, S., & Humphries, J. (1997). The origins and expansion of the male breadwinner family: The case of nineteenth-century Britain. *International Review of Social History*, 42(S5), 25–64. http://dx.doi.org/10.1017/S0020859000114786

Huenchuan, S. (2013). *Los derechos de las personas mayores*. Santiago de Chile, Chile: CEPAL. Retrieved from https://www.cepal.org/celade/noticias/documentosdetraba jo/8/51618/Derechos_PMayores_M2.pdf

Huenchuan, S. (2016). *Envejecimiento e institucionalidad pública en América Latina y el Caribe: conceptos, metodologías y casos prácticos*. Santiago, Chile: United Nations, Comisión Económica para América Latina y el Caribe (CEPAL).

Hutchens, G. (2016). *IMF managing director Christine Lagarde warns of demographic time-bomb. The Sunday Morning Herald*. Sydney, Australia. Retrieved from https://ww w.smh.com.au/business/the-economy/imf-managing-director-christine-lagarde-warns-of-demographic-timebomb-20160304-gnapv3.html.

International Labour Organization. (2019). *Informal employment (% of total non-agricultural employment) International Labour Organization, ILOSTAT database*. Retrieved from https://data.worldbank.org/indicator/SL.ISV.IFRM.ZS?locations=MX.

Jeppesen, H. (2016). *Amnesty's salil shetty: Human rights 'under attack'. Deutsche Welle (DW)*. Bonn, Germany. Retrieved from https://www.dw.com/en/amnestys-salil-shetty-human-rights-under-attack/a-19068608

Keck, M., & Sikkink, K. (1998). *Activists beyond borders: Advocacy networks in international politics*. Ithaca, NY: Cornell University Press.

Kennedy, D. (2002). The international human rights movement: Part of the problem. *Harvard Human Rights Journal*, 15, 101–126.

Kirk, D. (1996). Demographic transition theory. *Population Studies*, 50(3), 361–387. Retrieved from http://www.jstor.org/stable/2174639

Madrid, R. L. (2003). *Retiring the state: The politics of pension privatization in Latin America and beyond*. Stanford, CA: Stanford University Press.

Maloney, W. F. (2004). Informality revisited. *World Development*, 32(7), 1159–1178. http://dx.doi.org/10.1016/j.worlddev.2004.01.008

Martin, C., Rodríguez, D., & Brown, P. B. (2015). *Human rights of older people: Universal and regional legal perspectives*. New York, NY: Springer Publishing Company.

McCarthy, M. A. (2017). *Dismantling solidarity: Capitalist politics and American pensions since the new deal* (1st ed.). Ithaca, NY: Cornell University Press.

Mesa-Lago, C. (2004). An appraisal of a quarter-century of structural pension reforms in Latin America. *CEPAL Review*, 84, 57–81.

Mesa-Lago, C. (2008). *Reassembling social security: A survey of pensions and health care reforms in Latin America*. New York, NY: Oxford University Press.

Michoń, P. (2008). Familisation and defamilisation policy in 22 European countries. *Poznań University of Economics Review*, 8(1), 34–54. Retrieved from http://www.ebr.edu.pl/pub/2008_1_34.pdf

Montes-de-Oca, V., Paredes, M., Rodríguez, V., & Garay, S. (2018). Older persons and human rights in Latin America and the Caribbean. *International Journal on Ageing in Developing Countries*, 2(2), 149–164. Retrieved from https://www.inia.org.mt/wp-content/uploads/2018/09/2.2-8-Montes-de-Oca-edited.pdf

Montes de Oca Zavala, V. (2014). Cuidados y servicios sociales frente a la dependencia en el marco del envejecimiento demográfico en México. In S. Huenchuan, R. I. Rodríguez, B. L. C. D. A. Bárcena, & M. A. Mancera (Eds.), *Autonomía y dignidad en la vejez: Teoría y práctica en políticas de derechos de las personas mayores* (pp. 169–181). Mexico City: CEPAL.

Moyn, S. (2010). *The last utopia: Human rights in history*. Cambridge, MA: Belknap Press.

Newson, L., & Bourne, A. W. (2011). Financing social pensions in low- and middle-income countries. In *Pension watch: Briefing on social protection in old age* (Vol. 4). London, England: HelpAge International.

Nielsen, R. W. (2015). *Demographic transition theory contradicted repeatedly by Data*. Retrieved from http://arxiv.org/ftp/arxiv/papers/1510/1510.00471.pdf

Noonan, R. K. (1995). Women against the state: Political opportunities and collective action frames in Chile's transition to democracy. *Sociological Forum*, 10(1), 81–111. Retrieved from http://www.jstor.org/stable/684759

OAS. (2015a). *Inter-American convention for protect the human rights in older persons*. New York, NY: Organization of American States. Retrieved from http://www.oas.org/en/sla/dil/docs/inter_american_treaties_A-70_human_rights_older_persons.pdf

OAS. (2015b). *Inter-American convention on protecting the human rights of older persons (A-70)*. New York, NY: Organization of American Sates. Retrieved from http://www.oas.org/en/sla/dil/inter_american_treaties_A-70_human_rights_older_persons.asp.

OAS. (2017). *Inter-Averican convention on protecting the human rights of older persons (A-70)*. Washington, DC: Organization of American States. Retrieved from http://www.oas.org/en/about/who_we_are.asp

Orenstein, M. A. (2008). *Privatizing pensions: The transnational campaign for social security reform*. Princeton, NJ: Princeton University Press.

Orenstein, M. A. (2011). Pension privatization in crisis: Death or rebirth of a global policy trend? *International Social Security Review*, 64(3), 65–80. http://dx.doi.org/10.1111/j.1468-246X.2011.01403.x

Palier, B (Ed.). (2010). *A long goodbye to bismark? The politics of welfare reform in continental Europe*. Amsterdam, the Netherlands: Amsterdam University Press.

Piñera, J. (Fall/Winter 1995/96). Empowering workers: The privatization of social security in Chile. *Cato Journal*, 15(2–3), 155–156.

Posner, E. A. (2014). *The twilight of human rights law*. New York, NY: Oxford University Press.

Rodriguez-Pinzón, D., & Martin, C. (2003). The international human rights status of elderly persons. *American University International Law Review, 18*(4), 915–1008.

Rofman, R., Apella, I., & Vezza, E (Eds.). (2013). *Más allá de las pensiones contributivas: Catorce experiencias en América Latina* (82724 ed.). Buenos Aires: Banco Mundial.

Secretaría de Bienestar. (2019). *Programa para el bienestar de las personas adultas mayores.* Gobierno de México. Mexico City. Retrieved from https://www.gob.mx/bienestar/acciones-y-programas/programa-para-el-bienestar-de-las-personas-adultas-mayores.

Sidorenko, A., & Zaidi, A. (2018). International policy frameworks on ageing: Assessing progress in reference to the madrid international plan of action on ageing. *Journal of Social Policy Studies, 16*(1), 141–154. http://dx.doi.org/10.17323/727-0634-2018-16-1-141-154

Sikkink, K. (2017). *Evidence for hope: Making human rights work in the 21st century.* Princeton, NJ: Princeton University Press.

Snow, D. E., Burke Rochford, J., Worden, S. K., & Benford, R. D. (1986). Frame alignment processes, Micromobilization, and movement participation. *American Sociological Review, 51,* 464–481.

Strangio, S. (2017). *Welcome to the post-human rights world. Foreign Affairs.*Washington, DC. Retrieved from https://foreignpolicy.com/2017/03/07/welcome-to-the-post-human-rights-world/.

Tharoor, S. (1999/2000). Are human rights universal? *World Policy Journal, 16*(4), 1–6.

Torre, A. de la, & Rudolph, H. P. (2018). The troubled state of pension systems in Latin America. In *Global economy & development working paper 112.* Washington, DC: Brookings Institution. Retrieved from https://www.brookings.edu/wp-content/uploads/2018/03/working-paper_torre_rudolph_20182.pdf.

Turner, R. H. (1969). The theme of contemporary social movements. *British Journal of Sociology, 20,* 390–405.

United Nations. (1948). *Universal declaration of human rights.* Retrieved from https://www.un.org/en/universal-declaration-human-rights/index.html.

United Nations. (1982). *Report of the world assembly on aging.* New York, NY: Author. Retrieved from https://www.un.org/esa/socdev/ageing/documents/Resources/VIPEE-English.pdf

United Nations. (2002). *Report of the second world assembly on ageing. Madrid.* New York, NY: United Nations. Retrieved from https://documents-dds-ny.un.org/doc/UNDOC/GEN/N02/397/51/PDF/N0239751.pdf?OpenElement

Wada, T. (2006). Claim network analysis: How are social protests transformed into political protests in Mexico? In H. Johnston & P. Almeida (Eds.), *Latin American social movements: Globalization, democratization, and transnational networks* (pp. 95–111). New York, NY: Rowman & Littlefield Publishers, Inc.

Willmore, L. (2006). Universal age pensions in developing countries: The example of Mauritius. *International Social Security Review, 59*(4), 67–89.

Willmore, L. (2014). *Old age pensions in Mexico: Toward universal coverage*. Rochester, NY: Social Science Research Network. Retrieved from http://dx.doi.org/10.2139/ssrn.2383768

World Economic Forum. (2019). *Population, ageing and immigration: Germany's demographic question*. Retrieved from https://www.weforum.org/agenda/2017/04/population-ageing-and-immigration-germanys-demographic-question

Zaidi, B., & Morgan, S. P. (2017). The second demographic transition theory: A review and appraisal. *Annual Review of Sociology*, 43, 473–492. http://dx.doi.org/10.1146/annurev-soc-060116-053442

Index

Note: Page references followed by "*f*" denote figures

9 780826 143334